Praise for *The Hormone Fix*

"Hormones impact all aspects of your health. Master your hormones, master your health, master your life. It's never too late to thrive. This book is your guide to doing exactly that."
—Mark Hyman, MD, *New York Times* bestselling author of
The Blood Sugar Solution

"*The Hormone Fix* is a treasure trove of accurate and user-friendly information that all women who are suffering during menopause need to know and apply. It is written by an OBGYN who knows the territory both personally and professionally. I highly recommend this book."
—Christiane Northrup, MD, *New York Times* bestselling author of
The Wisdom of Menopause

"Dr. Anna Cabeca is a true innovator. She's also a powerful crusader for women's health. Her experiences help her to tell it like it is, but also to approach even the most delicate topics with warmth and compassion. *The Hormone Fix* is a perfect example of what happens when brains, heart, and fearless innovation come together. In other words, what happens when Anna Cabeca walks into the room!"
—JJ Virgin, triple-board certified nutrition expert and
New York Times bestselling author of *The Virgin Diet*

"This is an urgently needed book that every woman should read. *The Hormone Fix* provides clear, practical, and easy-to-follow steps that will correct hormone-related symptoms. Dr. Anna Cabecca has combined decades of practical experience and wisdom to provide a safe solution to health issues that women face today."
—Steven Masley, MD, FAHA, FACN, FAAFP, CNS,
author of *The Better Brain Solution*

"You'll want Dr. Cabeca's secrets to getting your sexy back! She shows you how to lose those last ten pounds, double your energy, and fall in love with yourself again, naturally."
—Robin Nielsen, CNC, BCHN

"Dr. Cabeca brings an incredible level of clarity to the task of optimizing hormone function—a task that has long proven a challenge for patients and clinicians alike. *The Hormone Fix* demystifies the complexities surrounding hormone function and interpreting laboratory tests. She then explores how the well-defined but often overlooked influences of environmental toxins as well as dietary choices affect hormone function. There is so much a woman can do to regain health through hormone balance, and Dr. Cabeca provides the road map."

—David Perlmutter, MD, *New York Times* bestselling author of *Grain Brain*

"Packed full of excellent information that's all based on the latest scientific research, *The Hormone Fix* makes the subject of hormone balance understandable and, even better, it makes achieving it doable! Dr. Cabeca's delicious Keto-Green recipes wisely point women toward a much more nutrient-dense way to do the popular keto diet."

—Leanne Ely, CNC, *New York Times* bestselling author and creator of SavingDinner.com

"Dr. Cabeca has cracked the code for weight loss. For many patients, going keto is not enough. Her brilliant wisdom and decades of experience helping women achieve wellness goals shines in this outstanding easy-to-read guide. Highly recommended."

—Ellie Campbell, DO, board certified in family medicine and integrative holistic medicine

"Dr. Anna Cabeca is a pioneer in women's health and natural ways to restore hormonal balance. In *The Hormone Fix*, she provides a concise road map to balanced hormones through deep healing and nutrition; her raw honesty in sharing her own journey makes the book even more impactful. I recommend it to all of my perimenopausal and menopausal women!"

—Angeli Maun Akey, MD, FACP, author of *Fine-Tune Your Hormone Symphony*

"Dr. Anna Cabeca is a pioneer in the field of women's menopausal health, and she brings her expertise into this fantastic book. Her book provides women with useful, impactful, and easy-to-implement solutions that will bring them back to pristine health. Every woman should have *The Hormone Fix* on her bookshelf and share it with her daughters."

—Isa Herrera, MSPT, CSCS, author of *Female Pelvic Alchemy* and founder of PelvicPainRelief.com

"Dr. Anna Cabeca is the authority on fixing women's hormones by using an innovative nutritional strategy that combines keto dieting, alkaline food choices, and lifestyle techniques that balance three key hormones. No one has put these pieces together until now. Follow Dr. Anna's program and experience rapid yet safe weight loss and resolution of your most nagging hormonal symptoms."

—Josh Axe, DNM, DC, CNS, author of *Keto Diet* and cofounder of Ancient Nutrition

"*The Hormone Fix* is a must-have resource for women who are struggling with hormone-related health challenges and want to get their lives back on track."

—Terry Wahls, MD, IFMCP, author of *The Wahls Protocol*

"Dr. Cabeca's Keto-Green eating plan is an incredible gift to women over forty. If you're struggling with weight gain, lagging energy, sleeplessness, and other hormone-related issues, this book is your road map back to better health!"

—Tess Masters, author of *The Perfect Blend*

"Dr. Anna Cabeca is an exciting innovator with a huge heart, always striving to improve the lives of women and their families. I can't wait to hear what she shares next."

—Rachel Hanfling, Executive Communications Trainer and creator of the Language of Leadership: The Results by Rachel System

"Dr. Anna Cabeca is the world-class expert you need to guide you through the challenging territory of menopause. If you're experiencing brain fog, vaginal dryness, weight gain, mood swings, or other symptoms, she has safe, natural solutions that truly work. So don't waste any more time suffering! Instead, read *The Hormone Fix,* and take back your life."

—Dr. Kellyann Petrucci, author *Dr. Kellyann's Bone Broth Diet*

"*The Hormone Fix* is a unique and comprehensive lifestyle approach to help with the myriad symptoms women must navigate during menopause. Dr. Cabeca's emphasis on reducing exposure to endocrine disruptors and on the importance of filling most of one's plate with healthy vegetables resonated with me."

—Felice Gersh, MD, author of *PCOS SOS: A Gynecologist's Lifeline to Naturally Restore Your Rhythms, Hormones, and Happiness*

"Whether you want to lose weight, sleep better, increase intimacy, or just wake up feeling excited about life, this book is an effective healing program tailored for women."

—Izabella Wentz, PharmD, FASCP

The Hormone Fix

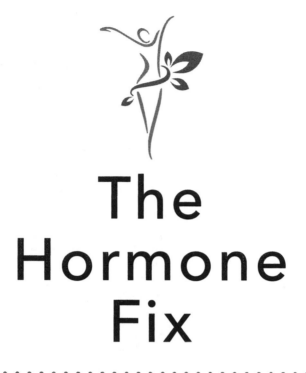

The Hormone Fix

· ·

BURN FAT NATURALLY, BOOST ENERGY,
SLEEP BETTER, AND STOP HOT FLASHES,
THE KETO-GREEN™ WAY

Anna Cabeca, DO, OBGYN, FACOG

BALLANTINE BOOKS

NEW YORK

No book can replace the diagnostic expertise and medical advice of a trusted physician. Please be certain to consult with your doctor before making any decisions that affect your health, particularly if you suffer from any medical condition or have any symptom that may require treatment.

The Hormone Fix is a work of nonfiction. Some names and identifying details have been changed.

Published in the United States by Ballantine Books, an imprint of Random House, a division of Penguin Random House LLC, New York.

BALLANTINE and the HOUSE colophon are registered trademarks of Penguin Random House LLC.

LIBRARY OF CONGRESS CATALOGING-IN-PUBLICATION DATA
Names: Cabeca, Anna, author.
Title: The hormone fix: burn fat naturally, boost energy, sleep better, and stop hot flashes, the keto-green way / Anna Cabeca, DO, OGBYN, FACOG.
Description: First edition. | New York: Ballantine Books, [2019] | Includes bibliographical references and index.
Identifiers: LCCN 2018051130 (print) | LCCN 2018054160 (ebook) | ISBN 9780525621652 (ebook) | ISBN 9780525621645 (hardback)
Subjects: LCSH: Menopause—Diet therapy—Popular works. | Ketogenic diet. | Menopause—Nutritional aspects. | Menopause—Diet therapy—Recipes. | BISAC: HEALTH & FITNESS / Diets. | HEALTH & FITNESS / Women's Health.
Classification: LCC RG186 (ebook) | LCC RG186 .C22 2019 (print) | DDC618.1/750654—dc23
LC record available at https://lccn.loc.gov/2018051130

Printed in the United States of America on acid-free paper

randomhousebooks.com

9 8 7 6 5 4

Book design by Diane Hobbing

I dedicate my book to my children.
I love you all so much and am so grateful for you.
You've given me laughter, life, and reason for being.

Foreword

I've known Dr. Anna Cabeca for more than fifteen years. I think of her as a true innovator, as well as a powerful crusader for women's health. Her experiences help her to tell it like it is, but also to approach even the most delicate topics with warmth and compassion.

But to me, Dr. Anna is more than just a brilliant physician; she's a dear friend. We've supported each other through some tough times. First, there was the tragic loss of her baby son, an experience that catapulted her into a personal crisis and then kicked off her search for the answers to hormonal imbalance that you'll find in these pages. Later, when my own son was in a brutal hit-and-run accident, Anna was one of the very first to reach out to me with words of hope and the sort of advice that can come only from someone who has been there.

Here's my point: No matter what you're facing, Dr. Anna is someone you want by your side! Her passion, sense of humor, and incredible intellect are evident after you've spent just a few minutes in her company.

One of my favorite things about Anna is how willing she is to challenge the status quo. Forget just thinking outside the box—this woman will create a door and escort you out of that box! Then she'll lead you to wide-open spaces where there are practical answers to the health issues that affect your life.

Case in point: When Anna lost her son, she didn't retreat from the world or try to push past the tragedy in order to keep life as it was before. Instead, she took her family on a yearlong, around-the-world healing journey, a trip that solidified her belief in the power and wisdom of integrative medicine. Her travels also introduced her to the superfood maca, which, in turn, inspired her to start a supplement company.

Aside from having extensive training, Anna is a generous, considerate woman, and she knows what it means to look out for others. I think that's what makes her so perfectly suited to taking a fresh look at dieting and piecing together the puzzle of women's health in a fresh new way.

I think we've been looking at diets all wrong. There is no one-size-fits-all version that will work for everyone for an entire lifetime. Instead, I believe that we should use diets therapeutically to achieve a specific result: identify food intolerances, lower fasting blood sugar, decrease autoimmune antibodies, lose body fat, etc. Then we can take the knowledge from that specific diet and use it to create an ongoing plan that is sustainable for the long term.

Every diet you go on should teach you new things about what works and what doesn't for your personal body chemistry and needs. And all of that is based on what is uniquely you—your genetics, your epigenetics, your lifestyle, your current state of health, your desired outcomes, and your readiness and motivation.

Dr. Anna created *The Hormone Fix* and her Keto-Green diet by following this very same process, first with herself and then with her patients. Big thinker that she is, she ingeniously took advantage of all the benefits of a ketogenic diet, while offsetting the downsides by incorporating the power of alkaline eating. I love that she also teaches you how to be your own personal health detective, how to prime your body for the process and then maximize the therapeutic effects. The result is a powerful program that you can personalize to help balance hormones and manage menopause for the long haul.

The Hormone Fix really is a perfect example of what happens when brains, heart, and fearless innovation come together. In other words, what happens when Dr. Anna Cabeca walks into the room!

—JJ Virgin, triple-board-certified nutrition
expert, *New York Times* bestselling author of
The Virgin Diet and *Sugar Impact Diet*

Contents

Introduction

Being a gynecologist and obstetrician for over two decades has given me the true honor and pleasure of taking care of generations of women at different stages of their lives, from their early teens through pregnancies, menopause, and well after. Wherever you are on that continuum, let's imagine it's you in my office. We're discussing your health and hormones and how you are honestly feeling. I close the door, and we sit down to talk after your annual Pap smear and physical exam. It's a vulnerable moment, I know. You've probably grappled with weight gain—maybe a little or a lot. Perhaps you've felt very forgetful, anxious, or moodier than before. Maybe you've started having hot flashes that go off like silent bombs inside you, or night sweats that make you want to sleep with the covers off, then on, then off again.

And what's your sex drive like? Is it fizzling out? Do you tire easily? Can't sleep a whole night, or wake up still tired? On top of everything else, do you no longer enjoy yourself or feel like your life isn't at all what it should be?

You might tell me about other symptoms. Perhaps you've been gaining weight, and you don't know why. Your relationships are fragmenting, along with your confidence. Thoughts may be swirling through your mind like: "Will I ever feel better? Am I just going downhill from here? Am I just going crazy? Or maybe there is something very wrong with me! Is it early Alzheimer's? Do I have cancer—thyroid, breast, ovarian? Is there something in my labs or my exam? Do I need a surgeon? Psychiatrist? Divorce attorney?"

Whoa, now!

I've sat with thousands of women in your situation, and I have communicated with many more thousands through my online interactive programs, including the two most popular, Magic Menopause and Sexual CPR, so I know that moment when you're ready to do anything. You want things fixed—now! But you may also have lost hope that it is still even possible. Take a deep breath. It is possible, it's not going to take a lot of time, and you're not alone. I assure you, you are a powerful woman, and you can turn things around fast.

I understand what's happening to you. You're struggling with the physical, mental, and emotional indignities of hormonal fluctuations and an ensuing "metabolic stall." The result: weight gain, hot flashes, night sweats, fatigue, insomnia, memory loss, hair loss, brain fog, irritability, diminished libido, discomfort during sex, pain, and more. Your body is winding down its reproductive machinery, and you feel like you're losing control—and losing your mind.

Too many women are resigned to accepting these changes, living unhappily with them, and muddling through for years to come. Many others will agree to be unnecessarily medicated for their symptoms. They're told this is normal or it's the best it's going to get. I know this because I often meet women after they have tried everything else and have gotten fed up with their medical care—yet still haven't given up hope.

And I also know what you're going through because I've been in this terrible place—twice!

My first experience with these hormonal changes occurred long before I approached menopause, and was triggered by a personal tragedy—my eighteen-month-old son died in a terrible and senseless accident. My insurmountable stress, deep grief, and subsequent depression thrust me into premature menopause and ovarian failure. My hormones were a mess. I was eighty pounds overweight. I couldn't lose a pound no matter how hard I tried. I started to lose my hair in clumps. My joints ached. At the time, I was the mother of three (two daughters and one stepdaughter), and I very much wanted another child. But because of my tragedy-induced premature hormonal changes, I was told by experts I could never get pregnant again and that I would have to live this way forever. I was devastated.

Mine was a health crisis that traditional medicine could not solve. I couldn't even solve it, despite being an Emory University–trained, board-certified ob-gyn and expert in functional medicine, plus a consultant in age management medicine. Dismissed by fellow doctors, I was informed that I would just have to live with infertility, weight gain, depression, fatigue, and hair loss. The only solution I was offered was antidepressants and sleeping pills. I felt shattered.

But I would not let myself stay broken.

I refused their options because I had seen my mother struggle under the weight of many medications, and I had to live for my daughters and search out solutions for myself. Survival alone was not enough. Eventually, by using an early version of the diet and lifestyle program I will share in this book, I lost those eighty pounds and went on to compete in a sprint triathlon (which is quite a personal accomplishment, because I hate to run!). My hormones leveled. My depression lifted, and I became someone who felt great all the time. Joyously, at age forty-one, I conceived a healthy baby girl. What traditional medicine said could not be done was done.

The second time happened in my late forties, more or less when most women expect to start transitioning away from monthly periods and into menopause. But just because it was expected didn't mean it was easy! My hormones mounted another attack on me. Weight gain that creeped to five pounds, ten pounds, then twenty pounds. More fatigue. Emotional volatility. Stress that made me feel like jumper cables were attached to my heart.

I didn't take this lying down. I went looking for answers and help. Unfortunately, I was again met with a "Well, this is normal" attitude and an ill-equipped medical system that could not, and would not, help. Can you relate? We're expected to tolerate and power through these disturbing changes, medicate them, or grin and bear them, right? No!

I knew what I had done previously to lose weight, fix my hormones, and overcome complete metabolic stall. I began to tinker with those same solutions again. It took me a lot of trial and error before I figured out the best way to reclaim my body, mind, and soul. I changed the way I ate. I changed lifestyle habits that were standing in my way. I tapped into my inner power and felt more contented and spiritually at peace.

Ultimately, I got myself back in tune. I was able to keep the creeping weight off, felt much more even-keeled—and really, like a younger version of myself. And that happy experience has inspired me to help other women, especially those struggling through hormonal chaos with nowhere to turn.

The book you are holding in your hands—*The Hormone Fix*—contains gems I learned through tragic personal experience, the day-to-day work of caring for more than ten thousand women in my medical clinic, and the coaching of a hundred thousand more online. Expressly for women (though the men in your life can follow it too), at its heart this is a breakthrough nutritional and lifestyle plan based on hard science, real people, and methods I use myself. It is so effective that you can lose up to a pound a day—without cravings, hunger, fatigue, or any of the side effects of other diets you may have tried. This unique program, along with supporting information on every single page, has the power to help you stay slim and sexy, feel more energetic, revive your libido, look and feel younger—and transform your life in ways you can't even yet imagine. It is the hope you've been looking for. I feel blessed to bring it to you now.

Not Your Average Doctor

As I hinted above, I did not create *The Hormone Fix* overnight and simply start putting patients on it. No, it took more than ten years of clinical work with real patients, exhaustive research and refinement, and most of all, personal experience and my own hormone hell.

But in many ways this program started with the needs of members of my own family. My mother had diabetes and heart disease. At one point, she was taking eleven prescription drugs and was in and out of the hospital. None of this saved her. She died at age sixty-seven after a heart valve replacement surgery. I was only thirty-one, in my residency at Emory University, and a new mom myself when she died. I was heartbroken, of course, and never accepted that her death had to be. I knew that there must be holistic answers to the malicious riddles of life-threatening diseases like hers. Finding them is what mattered to me then *and* now.

Also, my dad had diabetes. When doctors counted him out at age seventy-nine, saying he had led a "good life," I was incensed—and so was he. I helped him change his diet, added supplements and hormones, and took him off three prescription medicines. He went on to live another twelve good years.

Then there was my daughter Amanda—a smart, active, and articulate child, but a child who could not sit still. I wanted to help her, but I didn't want to do it with medication. I figured there must be a connection between what she was eating and how she behaved. I did an enormous amount of research into natural remedies; after all, this was my daughter. Based on what I learned, I decided she needed to have no more sugar, gluten, or caffeine-containing beverages. I reasoned that a change in diet, along with bioavailable B vitamins, fish oil, and other supplements would help Amanda become a healthy, active (not hyperactive) six-year-old. And they did.

Next came my own miracle of reversing premature menopause and becoming pregnant against the odds, as I've already described. Empowered by these personal experiences, I became fiercely determined to practice medicine more integratively with all my patients. I wanted to give them tools and information so that they could make informed decisions about their health and reclaim their natural ability to heal their own bodies. Often we are too quick to give our power over to pills or doctors, when our bodies have the ability to self-heal, given the right conditions and resources.

Hungrier for more knowledge on how to help people heal, I became a "professional student," attending conferences on integrative topics ranging from functional medicine to anti-aging and then applying this knowledge and clinical skills in my practice and fine-tuning it. I figured that if I could learn something that improved even one patient, it was worth my time. My greatest reward has been empowering women limited by their health to begin to enjoy life again. Ever since, I've been on a mission to assist as many women as I can to restore their health and begin leading long, healthy, loving, and fulfilling lives. It was too late to help my mom, but I could help others.

Whatever specific reason or symptom brought you to this book, I want you to thrive and become your most healthy, energetic, sexy, feminine, and vital self. We have so much to live for in these next wonderful stages of life—which is why we must take our health and power back and turn to lifestyle changes that will not only ease our discomfort and unhappiness but empower us to live out our best life with fun, love, and connection.

Now at age fifty-two, with a ten-year-old as well as three grown daughters, I want to live to be part of their children's lives, and to torment my kids well into my old age! I do not want to follow the path of my mom, suffering for years and then dying without ever having really known her grandkids and, worse, them not knowing her. Too many good women and men have gone down a path of unnecessary suffering, and I intend to put a stop to it. Enough is enough! You are powerful; you can do this.

Putting It All Together

The Hormone Fix features my short-term Keto-Green Quick Start Detox and my longer-term program, the Keto-Green Diet. Both help you improve your symptoms, diminish and even completely eliminate hot flashes, lose extra weight, get a clear mind, have glowing skin and hair, become connected, and, as a bonus, fully rejuvenate your life. Its associated lifestyle strategies will help lower your blood pressure, cholesterol, blood sugar, and weight in ways that standard medical care is just not able to accomplish. This is a program that saves lives.

With this in mind, here are some specifics you'll discover:

- How to lose up to a pound a day with my 10-Day Keto-Green Quick Start Detox. It is both hormone-fixing and fat-burning. Fair warning: the plan is a little stringent, but you will be eating delicious foods and experiencing energy that won't quit. You'll feel great while on it. The Quick Start is also an invaluable tool, not just something you'll do once. You can and should use it as a detox and cleanse periodically throughout the year for improved hormonal health. Go on it once a month, or at the start of each new season. Go back to the Quick Start if your weight starts creeping up or if you need to slim down quickly for a special occasion. The Quick Start is a plan you can enjoy anytime, for any reason.

- How to continue your success with my 21-Day Keto-Green Diet—an eating guide that can be used forever (and for which I've given you three weeks' worth of options and ideas). It provides tasty, filling options for meals that help balance your hormones naturally—and thus reduce or eliminate hot flashes, cravings, depression and anxiety, low sex drive, premature aging, thinning hair, aches and pain, and other symptoms that may be wrecking your life and self-esteem.
- Why this plan works for a wide range of life stages—perimenopause, menopause, and postmenopause—and even for the men in your life who may be facing their own weight, blood sugar, and hormonal issues.
- How to identify the underlying causes of your symptoms, track your progress over time, completely reverse what has been sabotaging your efforts, and take back your life.
- Why you will dramatically improve your memory, focus, and motivation by restoring brain-nurturing chemicals to more youthful levels. When you go Keto-Green, you'll experience energized enlightenment and feel mentally and spiritually alive.
- Which revitalizing lifestyle strategies help fix your hormones. It isn't all about diet. Hydration becomes crucial. So does sleeping well, exercising, enjoying healthy relationships, managing stress, and living with peace and purpose.

With *The Hormone Fix,* you will be well on your way to slimming down, feeling more energized, and enjoying clearer thinking. I can see you smiling now. You're getting it. No more powering through nagging symptoms of fluctuating hormones. No more feeling tyrannized by stress.

Believe me, I know how overwhelming life can feel sometimes. But don't give up on yourself. You are about to tap into unexpected energy levels and enhanced intimacy. In short, you'll be creating the very best you! I truly believe every woman deserves and can achieve a vibrantly healthy life filled with love and happiness. And that means you!

Menopause is not a disease that needs some kind of cure; it is a natural transition to be approached as a new type of freedom and personal power. This is a beautiful, important time in your life—a time to look forward, chart a new course, and enjoy what can be the most exciting decades of your life. You are about to journey in a new direction, toward health, happiness, and wholeness, and I'll be with you every step of the way.

Sound good? Then let's begin.

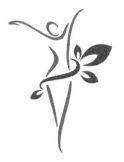

PART ONE

· ·

Hormonal Harmony

Chapter 1

What's Going On with My Hormones?

Deborah, age sixty-two, was really struggling when she came to me. "I just don't feel right," she said. "My energy is down, and my weight is up. No matter what I do, I can't seem to fix my energy or lose the weight."

She felt sad all the time, and her moods swung all over the place. "I'll be somewhere and suddenly burst into tears or anger for no reason."

Deborah suffered through many sleepless nights too, unless she used sleep aids, but even with those, she did not wake feeling rested. Her hot flashes were so severe that her body felt like a steam vent, and she'd perspire all over.

"This has been going on so long, I can't remember the last time I felt well. I'm beginning to think that my life is over," she said.

Rita, forty-four, was in a state of physical and mental chaos. "I have unbelievable hot flashes, brain fog, and dry skin. I am emotional all the time and piling on weight. Hair is growing on my face and I'm losing it from my head! I feel like I am losing my identity, because I no longer feel feminine." Hormone changes were hitting home, and hitting hard. "It is hard to see a light at the end of the tunnel when your body is changing," she said. "I try to tell myself it won't last forever. But what will I be like after menopause? I'm too young to feel this way."

At age fifty-three, Tina had to drag herself out of bed in the morning.

Her eyes stung from crying all the time, and she was totally exhausted. "I have a rough time losing pounds, no matter how hard I diet. Nothing works." She sighed. "I look awful, feel awful, and have no desire to be intimate with my husband. I'm not living my life. I can't cope with feeling this way forever."

In my twenty-plus years in medicine, I've met many women like Deborah, Rita, and Tina. I've heard their stories and their pleas. They are plagued by hormonal imbalances, which may have begun around age thirty-five when levels of progesterone, a crucial reproductive hormone, begin to decrease. Estrogen, vital to numerous functions including bone protection and brain function, starts falling off in your forties and fifties, increasing your risk for osteoporosis and other problems. Testosterone also begins to decline in midlife, and dehydroepiandrosterone (DHEA) starts decreasing in our twenties. A deficit of DHEA contributes to loss of sex drive, vaginal dryness, osteoporosis, and lots more. Altogether, these and other hormonal pendulum swings create a perfect storm for menopausal miseries, including weight gain, mood swings, and crashing libido—and what is worse, a sense that you no longer know or like your body or yourself.

Deborah, Rita, and Tina are women who were scared, troubled, and beaten down by seemingly out-of-control symptoms brought on by declining hormones and advancing age. They felt miserable and hopeless. And obviously, that is a bad place to be.

Although these women had different experiences, their symptoms and problems were resolved through a common route: the Hormone Fix, a program that I developed over years of testing and have now been using with clients for years. It is a practical way to transition into and from times of fluctuating hormones while minimizing or eliminating many of the miseries and ensuing critical health conditions. It helps you gently change your lifestyle, while enhancing your life. It leads you to embrace the kind of positive habits that will start transforming your body, even in the midst of the often confusing but natural and beautiful life stage of menopause.

Deborah, for example, decided she was ready to change. She got serious with my Keto-Green Diet and lifestyle. Within weeks, her troublesome, life-limiting symptoms of hot flashes and sleeplessness practically vanished. She lost ten pounds, two inches from her waist, and three inches from her hips.

Rita is now loving life again. Her mind is clearer, her moods are better, and she has more energy than ever. The excess fat began melting off. Her symptoms of early menopause disappeared. She loved it when the attendant at her usual service station remarked that she looked like she was eighteen. She'd regained bounds of youthful energy too!

Tina lost twenty-eight pounds with the Keto-Green Diet and lifestyle and pared inches off her figure—something she had not been able to do in a very long time. Her cravings for fattening foods were eliminated. And she was back to her energetic self—and a loving, vibrant sex life with her husband, for which she is ever grateful.

Their renewed health and success can be yours too.

Hormones 101

Each day, more than 150 chemicals called hormones run through your body. They act as chemical messengers, orchestrating an intricate symphony of messages telling your organs what your brain wants them to do. Hormones are really exciting because they influence many bodily functions, including metabolism, reproduction, blood sugar levels, blood pressure, energy levels, kidney function, sleep patterns, aging, appetite, sex drive, and more.

Hormones are secreted by organs called endocrine glands, which include the pituitary, thyroid, hypothalamus, ovaries, and testes. Other organs and tissues emit hormones too—namely, the kidneys, heart, small intestine, and even your own fat tissue.

Your body employs a feedback system to keep hormones in precise balance. That is, when one hormone is present in abnormally high or low levels, the body sets in motion a chain of reactions that balances the system. You can think of this feedback system as being like the thermostat in your house. You set it at a desired temperature, and when the internal thermometer senses an increase or decrease of a few degrees, it immediately sends a signal to turn on the air conditioner or heater to cool or heat up the room.

In your body, the control mechanism is the pituitary gland. It sits at the base of your brain and detects changes in the levels of these chemicals in the body. Sensing changes, the pituitary increases or decreases its gland-specific stimulating hormones to bring the body back in balance. Numerous factors can throw off this delicate balance, including a lack of nutrients, aging, diseases, alcohol and drugs, sleep problems, and stress, both physical and emotional.

How Hormones Change at Various Life Stages

The beautiful and natural biological patterns in your life are governed by your hormones. When you were a teenager, the arrival of your menstrual cycle opened the door to your womanhood. During each menstrual cycle, the pituitary gland releases follicle-stimulating hormone (FSH) and luteinizing hormone (LH). They are responsible for the development of follicles (cells that contain immature eggs, known as ova). They also produce estrogen and progesterone, which stimulate the uterus to build up its lining with extra blood and tissue. This process thickens and cushions the uterine walls in preparation for pregnancy.

About once a month, a tiny egg departs from one of the ovaries (ovulation) and heads to the uterus through one of the fallopian tubes. If the egg is fertilized by a sperm cell, it settles in the uterus and attaches to its cushiony walls, where it slowly develops into a baby. If the egg isn't fertilized, it won't affix to the uterine wall. When this happens, the uterus sloughs off its extra lining. The blood, tissue, and unfertilized egg exit the uterus, passing through the vagina on the way out of the body. This is your period. For the next few decades of your life, it will arrive as regularly as your bank statement, unless you get pregnant.

Hormonally, in your twenties you've shed the chrysalis of your teen years and spread your adult wings. You're packing on bone mass, developing lean muscle, and pumping out estrogen, progesterone, testosterone, DHEA, and other reproductive hormones at peak levels. Your monthly cycle is a reminder of your fertility.

By the time you reach your midthirties, your metabolism starts slowing down. It gets a little easier to gain extra pounds, even if you stick to the same exercise program and nutritional diet of your twenties. Your body fat is about 25 percent, and your hips and thighs are spreading a bit.

In both your twenties and thirties, your sex drive is likely high, thanks to elevated sex hormones. And that's as it should be. You want to be nice and frisky in your primary childbearing years.

Each of us is born with a finite number of eggs, and those eggs are aging with us. Therefore, and naturally, as you get closer to your forties, your fertility begins to drop sharply. You'll also have a decline in the level of estrogen in your blood, which shrinks the amount of collagen and elastin in your skin, reducing its firmness and springiness. You might notice a few wrinkles here and there when you look in the mirror.

Your forties are the transitional years between childbearing and menopause, and therefore the decade in which you go through peri-menopause (though perimenopause can last anywhere from five to fifteen years). The first main reproductive hormone to start its descent is progesterone, followed by estrogen and others. You'll have symptoms that foreshadow menopause: missed periods, PMS, breakthrough bleeding, palpitations, migraines, hot flashes, vaginal dryness, insomnia, and anxiety, among others. During perimenopause, some of you may feel like your body isn't your own anymore, like something is seriously wrong. Do migraines mean a brain tumor? Do palpitations signal a heart attack? No . . . it is just nature messing with your hormonal balance.

I tell my patients that if you hate your husband or partner only two weeks out of the month, it is your hormones, not your spouse or partner. This whole cascade of crazy hormones at this time often results in a lack of self-care—which, in turn, causes resentment toward yourself and loved ones. At no time in your life is self-care more important than when you are approaching the transition of menopause. Take care of yourself now, and you will cement habits that will serve you well into your golden years.

Next comes menopause. Even though we often speak of menopause as the part of your life in which your period has ceased, it's actually technically defined as the date twelve months after your last period. Thereafter, you are actually postmenopausal. When I use the words "menopause" and "menopausal" in this book, I am referring to the entire transitional time before and after menopause. The average age of menopause for most women is approximately fifty-one, but much younger if you smoke. Menopause is when your body is shutting down its reproductive capacity, drastically affecting just about every organ.

Hormonally, what does menopause look like? Your estrogen levels, which fluctuated wildly during perimenopause (the time prior to menopause), drop 75 percent or more from their peak. For some, this major change is easy and trouble-free, with few problems and manageable symptoms. For others, there are unpleasant, often debilitating symptoms like hair loss, acne, aches and pains, crashing fatigue, and weight gain. As estrogen falls off, fat shows up in certain areas—the tummy, thighs, butt, chin, and under-eye area.

Sexually, menopause presents a mixed bag. The loss of estrogen makes the vaginal walls less elastic, resulting in dryness, loss of lubrication, decreased sensation, and sometimes pain during intercourse. The labia shrink a bit too, exposing more of the clitoris, which can become less sensitive with age. (I'll give you strategies in Chapter 9 on how to improve these vaginal issues.)

Meanwhile, you might look in the mirror or at your hands and see that your skin is thinner and more crepey. At fifty, you might have gray hair—a lot or a little. It might also be noticeably thinner and drier than it used to be.

With the onset of menopause, you may lose bone mass quite rapidly. The declines in estrogen, progesterone, testosterone, and DHEA cause a change in the absorption of skeletal calcium. You can help prevent this with vitamin D and K supplementation, strength training, and eating a high-mineral and alkaline diet. If you haven't been doing most of this, you face a high risk of developing osteoporosis.

Despite these changes, menopause is not a disease—far from it. It's another natural stage in your life, when your hormones are in flux once again.

As menopause ends, you enter postmenopause—which can actually be quite liberating, a new place of centeredness, and a potentially very rewarding phase of life. You begin to reassess your life and goals. You're more inclined to say, "What shall I do in the next season of my life?"

After all, you do have a lot of living left to do! You still have dreams to fulfill—perhaps an entrepreneurial idea, a trip around the world, a volunteer commitment to your favorite cause, a run for office. You are more independent than ever and can move in the direction of new hopes and goals—especially if you have your health.

A favorite quote of mine is: "When you have your health, you have a million wishes, when you don't, you only have one wish . . . and that is to have health."

Despite your continued decline in metabolism, you don't gain as much weight when you are postmenopausal because your appetite may decrease. But any extra pounds added to your waist in your forties and fifties have increased your risk of high blood pressure, heart disease, memory loss, and diabetes (the extra weight around the midsection can also be a sign of insulin resistance). It is not too late, however, to implement healthier practices in your life.

Happily, the probability of living well into your postmenopausal years is greater than ever before—and growing all the time. Modern women could reasonably expect to enjoy a vibrant quality of life at least into their eighties—a gain of thirty years of life compared to women born in the 1800s! Wiser now, you can enjoy the life that you worked so hard to create, while being able to educate, inspire, and instruct those around you and the generations that follow.

Each stage of your life can be a doorway to discovery, where you can find out what gives you joy, recognize what you are grateful for, and explore opportunities to fulfill your dreams, even the ones yet unrealized. As you leave one journey, you begin another, not with a sense of regret, but with a new appreciation of change and what the future holds.

The Three Magic Hormones and How They Work in Your Body

You might think that estrogen, progesterone, testosterone, and other sex hormones are the major players during these life changes. But they are not. Specifically, when it comes to menopause, the three hormones that we need to be concerned with—the ones that are the major players—are insulin, cortisol, and oxytocin. When these are balanced, all the other hormones in your body fall into line. My program—including my unique Keto-Green Diet—focuses on these key hormones.

Each hormone is intimately involved in how you feel, how you think, and how you look. If you feel less than whole as your body goes through its natural age-related changes, it is likely because you have an imbalance of these hormones. Correcting the imbalances through diet and lifestyle can restore you not only to your previous healthy self but to a younger, sexier, and fitter version of yourself that you and others really love.

Insulin and the Keto-Green Diet

Insulin is a major hormone, and it can affect many other hormones, including the sex hormones (estrogen, progesterone, and testosterone). So when it is unbalanced, other hormones go out of kilter too.

Women can become insulin-resistant as they approach menopause mostly because their bodies can no longer deal with high amounts of carbohydrates, nor with snacking. Which means that the carbs you once ate—even healthy ones like fruits, whole grains, potatoes, or brown rice—will affect your waistline. When cells can't soak up the extra glucose because of insulin resistance, the liver has to deal with it by converting it into fat.

Insulin resistance lurks beneath many of the most common symptoms you experience during menopause: hot flashes, fatigue, difficulty concentrating, and weight gain. All of these are early symptoms of insulin resistance, but we often don't make the connection, because no one has pointed it out to us.

On top of all this, insulin resistance is closely linked to many other serious health problems such as diabetes, polycystic ovary syndrome (PCOS), high blood pressure, abnormal cholesterol, breast cancer, and endometrial cancer, and has been implicated in Alzheimer's disease.

My combination of keto and alkaline eating—the Keto-Green Diet—helps regulate insulin and reverse insulin resistance in one important way: it shifts you into ketosis, which restores your body to an insulin-sensitive state.

The ketogenic component of the diet works by keeping the body's carbohydrate stores almost empty. Your body starts burning its own body fat for energy, helping you lose weight quickly. It will also burn fat that you're consuming through your diet, assuming you are eating healthy fats (not trans fats, for example).

When you're insulin sensitive, all sorts of metabolic miracles happen. You stay slimmer and fitter. You lower your risk of cardiovascular disease, Alzheimer's disease, and dementia. You tend to not have hot flashes or night sweats. You rebuild your bone health so that you're at less risk for frailty and osteoporosis. Cravings become a distant memory. And you feel, look, and act healthy and energized.

Cortisol and the Keto-Green Way

Cortisol is the key stress hormone and one of the lifesaving hormones. It is an immediate responder in times of danger and stress. Following a stressful event, your adrenal glands pour out cortisol. Cortisol boosts the amount of blood sugar available for fuel and revs up your heart rate so you can fight off or escape a threat, or otherwise deal with the stress.

After the danger passes, cortisol also functions as the "cleanup crew" to lower inflammation, a damaging side effect of the stress response. Cortisol, then, serves as the body's natural anti-inflammatory hormone.

So all the intentions of this hormone are good. But often cortisol stays elevated in the body for too long due to chronic, unresolved stress (real or perceived). Over time, its efforts to reduce inflammation stall and suppress immunity, leading to an increased susceptibility to colds and other illnesses. Chronically elevated cortisol can actually damage our body. It increases acidity, throws our gut flora out of whack, and causes "leaky gut," when the gut becomes so permeable that substances and nutrients actually seep out through the intestinal wall. In short, cortisol knocks our bodies out of balance. It becomes the Rocky Balboa of hormones!

Chronic high cortisol can also lead to rapid aging, depression, adrenal fatigue, feelings of loneliness and burnout—all due to a domino-like sequence of events. Just look at photographs of any president before taking office and after leaving office, and you can see the effects of stress on aging in just four to eight years.

So, what's happening? First, the presence of elevated cortisol activates the paraventricular nucleus (PVN) in the brain—a control center regulating stress, metabolism, growth, reproduction, immunity, and other functions. Second, the PVN tells the adrenal glands, which produce cortisol and other hormones, to stop making so much cortisol because its mass production is frying the body. If this cascade of events goes unchecked, inflammation then takes over. And that segues into more rapid aging, emotional problems, and other bodily disasters. Sadly, as we get older, there is less automatic regulation of cortisol. It can continue to circulate, increasing our risks for dementia, heart disease, osteoporosis, metabolic syndrome, cancer, and more.

Also, the secretion of high amounts of cortisol robs your body of DHEA, progesterone, estrogen, and testosterone. The net effects are increased glucose production, decreased lean muscle production, imbalances of estrogen and testosterone, low sex drive and desire, and burnout.

Chronic elevation of cortisol can pack on pounds in three ways. One way has to do with visceral fat cells (the ones in our abdomen and around our vital organs). Cortisol triggers a fat-storing enzyme in those fat cells, causing many of us to put on more belly fat. Belly fat cells seem to attract cortisol too. They have four times as many cortisol receptors as regular fat cells.

A second way in which cortisol is involved in weight gain has to do with the blood sugar/insulin problem. When cortisol hangs around 24/7, it raises your blood sugar levels and keeps them high. This creates insulin resistance. Glucose can't get into cells the way it normally would. Eventually it is stored as fat.

The third connection is cortisol's effect on appetite and cravings for high-calorie foods. When cortisol levels rise, you're likely to have food cravings. In women, those cravings tend to be strongest for carbs, especially sweets when you're feeling sad or moody, and crunchy, salty chips when you're feeling stressed and irritated.

During menopause, the body's reduced ability to control that spiking cortisol (with its effect of reduced insulin sensitivity) is what contributes to hot flashes, night sweats, weight gain, mood swings, anxiety, insomnia, and more.

Cortisol is directly related to weight gain. Switching to more alkaline foods and lifestyle habits curtails levels of cortisol, which is one reason that both actions help you lose body fat. There is a definite and positive connection between following an alkaline diet, lowering cortisol, and burning fat. If you want all that—and I know you do—you've got to stay in an alkaline environment. To make sure, you can easily check your urine pH (more on how to do that on page 30).

BALANCED HORMONES, BALANCED BODY

SYMPTOMS OF EXCESS ESTROGEN	SYMPTOMS OF LOW ESTROGEN
Mood swings	Mental fogginess or forgetfulness
Irritability	Depression
Depression	Anxiety
Irregular periods	Moodiness
Hot flashes	Hot flashes
Vaginal dryness	Night sweats
Water retention	Fatigue
Weight gain in hips, thighs, and tummy	Decreased libido
Poor sleep quality	Dry eyes, skin, and vagina
Decreased libido	Loss of skin radiance
Headaches	Sagging breasts
Fatigue	Pain during intercourse
Short-term memory loss	Weight gain
Poor concentration	Increased back and joint pain
Thinning of scalp hair	Heart palpitations
Dry, thin, wrinkly skin	Headaches
Increased facial hair	Gastrointestinal discomfort
Bone mineral loss	Poor sleep quality
Osteoporosis	
Aches and pains	

SYMPTOMS OF EXCESS PROGESTERONE	SYMPTOMS OF LOW PROGESTERONE
Increased insulin resistance	Luteal phase defects (abnormal endometrial development)
21-hydroxylase deficiency (a short supply of an enzyme needed to convert cholesterol into cortisol)	Infertility and ovulation problems
Increased activity of lipoprotein lipase (an enzyme that increases fat storage)	Breast tenderness
	Depression
Loss of muscle tissue and muscle strength	Anxiety
	Fatigue
Decreased production of growth hormone	Poor concentration
	Endometriosis
High cortisol levels in the blood	Fibrocystic breasts
Sugar cravings	PMS/mood swings
Lower calorie expenditure	PCOS
Weight gain	Headaches
Estrogen deficiency symptoms (see above)	Fibroids
	Water retention and bloating
	Weight gain
	Breast and uterine cancer
	Cold body temperature
	Menstrual flow changes
SYMPTOMS OF TOO MUCH TESTOSTERONE OR DHEA	**SYMPTOMS OF TOO LITTLE TESTOSTERONE OR DHEA**
Acne	Decreased libido
Hair growth	Early senility
Aggression	Memory problems
Temporary hair loss	Reduced mental power
PCOS	Poor concentration
Infertility	Moodiness
Diabetes	Depression
Heart disease risk	Fatigue and weakness
Possibly poor prognosis in breast cancer	Passive attitude
	Irritability
	Less interest in normal activities
	Hypochondria

Oxytocin and the Keto-Green Way

Produced by the hypothalamus and secreted from the pituitary gland and other tissues, including the heart, uterus, and ovaries, oxytocin is my favorite hormone—the powerful hormone of love, bonding, and connection. It's the hormone that floods us during childbirth as we cradle our newborn. It also surges with orgasm, laughter, play, hugging, caressing your pet, and giving. It's an anti-aging hormone too.

Physiologically, oxytocin and cortisol have a love-hate relationship. They oppose each other. They are like two boxers in a ring, or the two kids on a seesaw. When one goes up, the other is forced to go down. I know this firsthand. The chronic stress and PTSD I endured from losing my son triggered the cortisol-oxytocin disconnect and made me unconsciously shun the things and people I loved. Simply put, I walked away because cortisol won. There is a definite physiology behind all this—you're not going crazy! If you ever experience burnout, emotional disconnection, or withdrawal from things and people you love, it is probably due to cortisol knocking oxytocin down.

Thankfully, oxytocin helps counterbalance cortisol's negative effects. That's why I sometimes say that you can "hug your belly fat away."—loving hugs are a great way to produce lots of oxytocin.

But wait, there's more! Oxytocin also helps regulate body weight and appetite. This makes sense when you remember the early stages of falling in love and having no appetite, right? In 2008, Japanese researchers demonstrated that if you take a mouse and knock out the oxytocin receptors on its cells, the mouse becomes obese, even without eating any more food than it usually does. Another study, reported in 2013, showed that if you give humans or mice extra oxytocin, the hormone prevents insulin resistance and triggers weight loss.

All of this adds up to the fact that there is a strong connection between oxytocin and eating. Oxytocin is very involved in satiety—the happy feeling of being full and satisfied after a meal. When you eat, various hormones are stimulated, including insulin, leptin, and cholecystokinin (CCK). As digestion begins, leptin and CCK signal the brain via the vagus nerve, the neural "highway" that runs up and down the trunk of your body and shuttles hunger and appetite impulses between your brain and your gut. In response, the hypothalamus (the appetite control center in the brain) releases oxytocin, which then helps produce that happy, full feeling in your tummy. Suddenly you're less hungry.

The reason oxytocin is an anti-aging hormone is that it increases cellular regeneration and health, plus prevents microbes from invading cells. You'll learn more about this wonderful hormone in Chapter 11.

Though there are not specific foods that help release oxytocin, research does show that chronic sugar intake reduces the amount of oxytocin that your body makes in response to food. So eating too much sugar suppresses oxytocin in your body. That's not good for weight control and is another reason why the Keto-Green Diet is low in sugar.

HORMONES, YOUR NEUROTRANSMITTERS, AND DIET

Neurotransmitters are powerful chemical messengers, just like hormones, and their levels are affected by hormonal imbalances. So when neurotransmitters are out of balance, this affects mood, cognition, attitude, coping skills, energy, sleep, overall health, and more.

Serotonin and Estrogen

Serotonin is the relaxing and calming neurotransmitter. It makes us feel good. When estrogen falls, levels of serotonin drop. As a result, we tend to feel moodier, easily irritated, and our appetite increases. What you eat can help this imbalance. That's because certain gut bacteria help boost brain levels of serotonin—so you want to eat plenty of probiotic rich foods, such as pickles, sauerkraut, yogurt with active cultures, and kefir. These foods promote healthy gut bacteria, which in turn increase serotonin. The spice turmeric, a well-known anti-inflammatory, also prolongs the activity of serotonin in the brain. Foods containing the amino acid tryptophan such as turkey, dairy, dates, and sunflower seeds, to name a few, and foods with high levels of omega-3 fatty acids, such as cold-water fish, flaxseed oil, and walnuts, are also thought to boost serotonin levels.

Dopamine and Testosterone

Dopamine is a powerful neurotransmitter that affects pleasure and motivation. High levels of dopamine give you enthusiasm and drive. Falling levels are linked to a sense of emptiness, sadness, irritation, and boredom. When dopamine is released, it triggers the production of testosterone, which is critical for sex drive in both men and women. To ensure a steady production of dopamine—and higher testosterone—you need to supply your brain with the nutrient building blocks of dopamine. One important building block is phenylalanine, found in beets, edamame, nuts, eggs, dairy, and meat. If you really need a quick mood boost, chocolate can bump up dopamine and serotonin. This is because it contains anandamide-like molecules, a fatty acid that acts like the active substance in marijuana.

GABA and Progesterone

Gamma-aminobutyric acid (GABA) gives your brain the peace and calm it needs. Progesterone acts on GABA receptors in the brain, but as progesterone declines with age, so does GABA. You're then prone to anxiety, depression, and poor sleep. Fortunately, there are GABA-boosting foods that can help counter this imbalance: cherry tomatoes, kefir (also a probiotic food), shrimp, green tea, lemon balm, ashwaganda, and any food high in omega-3 fats, such as salmon. GABA supplements taken at night can also be used to promote deeper sleep if needed.

Chapter 2

Where Are You Now? Test, Don't Guess!

You are beginning a beautiful, healing journey—all at a time when your hormones are fluctuating wildly. You know your destination: to have optimal health and longevity, be in shape, get back in the swing of sexual desire, energize yourself, and be free of hot flashes, night sweats, bad moods, brain fog, and other symptoms. In short, you want to feel better fast! So before we dive into my program, I want you to take a little time to find out where you are right now—in terms of your hormones, health, and emotions.

Toward that end, you'll take a series of eye-opening self-tests that:

- Decipher your levels of key hormones
- Identify symptoms that help point to the underlying causes of illness
- Assess your sexual and pelvic health
- Check how positive you are about yourself, your life, and your future
- Measure your waist and hip circumference
- Measure ketones and pH of your urine

These tests provide valuable information that even expensive blood tests can't tell you. My patients and the women in my online Magic

Menopause program love to test and retest themselves. The reason is that they see quantifiable progress. A typical example is Joanie. She was in great health until her second son was born. From there, she spiraled downhill with all sorts of hormonal imbalances and resulting symptoms. Joanie took my Medical Symptom Toxicity Questionnaire (one of the self-tests below) and scored 82. Unlike the tests you took in school, a high score is bad. The lower your score, the better! A score of 82 indicated that she had a lot of negative health issues going on in her body. But after one month of following my program, she retested and scored 32—a remarkable change. What she saw on paper mirrored how she felt. Joanie told me, "I feel like I have my healthy body back for the first time in twenty years."

My hope is that you will feel encouraged and inspired by using these tracking tools and seeing your own numbers go down. Having your own unique baseline information is important so you can see your changes over time. You may be amazed at your starting scores! But you'll be so excited to see your progress. Taking time to assess yourself will make sure you aren't overlooking anything—plus it helps you fine-tune and manage your progress as you implement healthy changes. I always say: *What is measured gets managed.*

You'll notice that I have reprinted the following checklist and tests in the back of the book so that you can more easily tear them out and really use them. In addition to testing at the onset of the program, I recommend that you test again after one month and after two months. (See dranna.com/resources.)

Hormonal Review of Symptoms Checklist

This is a helpful checklist that shows you what is likely happening to your key hormone levels, based on a variety of symptoms. It helps you see the linkages among all sorts of hormones.

Look at each symptom, listed in the far-left column. Then rate each symptom on a scale from 0 to 3 (0 = no symptoms; 1 = mild; 2 = moderate; 3 = severe). Record your rating in the far-right column under Symptom Score.

Compare your Symptom Score with what is going on with your hormones. For example, let's say you rated your hot flashes as a 3 (severe). Checking the Hormonal Relationship column, you see that your estrogen levels may be going up or down (↑ ↓E); your progesterone levels are declining (↓P); and your testosterone levels are declining too (↓T).

This scoring system is not quite as accurate as any blood test—but you don't have to pay for it. I'm not saying blood tests aren't valuable; they are, and they have their place, especially for fine-tuning hormonal balance. Just the same, this test gives you an accurate snapshot of where you are right now. Retake it after a month and after two months, and you will be surprised and delighted to see improvements not only in black and white, but also in how you look and feel.

Date_____

SYMPTOM	HORMONE RELATIONSHIP	SYMPTOM SCORE
Anxiety	↑E ↓P ↓T ↑C↓TH	
Arthritis	↓T ↓P	
Bladder symptoms	↓E ↓T	
Breakthrough bleeding	↓P	
Breast tenderness	↑E ↓P	
Constipation	↓TH	
Cramps or painful periods	↓P ↑P	
Decreased ability to play sports	↓T ↓TH	
Decreased enjoyment of life	↑E ↓P ↓T	
Decreased sex drive	↑ ↓E ↓P ↓T ↑ ↓C ↓TH	
Decreased strength or endurance	↓T ↓TH	
Decreased work performance	↓E ↓T ↓P ↓TH	
Depression	↑ ↓P ↑C ↓E ↑ ↓T ↓TH	
Dry skin/hair	↓E ↓TH	
Fatigue	↑P ↓TH ↓T ↑ ↓C ↑ ↓E	
Fibrocystic breasts	↑E ↓P	
Fluid retention	↑E ↓P	

Hair loss	↑T ↑↓TH ↑↓E ↑↓P ↑C	
Harder to reach climax	↓T ↓E ↓P	
Headaches	↑↓E ↑↓P ↓T ↑C ↓TH	
Heavy/irregular menses	↑E ↓P	
Hot flashes	↑↓E ↓P ↓T	
Irritability	↑E ↑↓P ↑T ↓C	
Loose stools	↑C ↑TH	
Loss of memory	↑↓E ↑↓P ↓T ↑C ↓TH	
Mood swings	↑E ↓P	
Night sweats	↑↓C ↓E	
Sleep disturbance	↑↓T ↓P ↓E ↑C	
Stomach pain	↑↓C	
Vaginal dryness	↓E ↓T	
Weakness, muscular	↓T ↓P	
Weight gain	↑E ↓P ↓TH	
Weight loss	↑C ↑TH	

Key: E = estrogen / P = progesterone / T = testosterone / C = cortisol / TH = thyroid

Record your total points: _____

Medical Symptom Toxicity Questionnaire

This assessment identifies symptoms that help point to the underlying causes of possible illness.

Using the point scale below, rate each of the following symptoms based on your symptoms over the last thirty days. For each symptom category, total your points.

Finally, add up the totals from each category to come up with your grand total.

POINT SCALE

0 = Never or almost never have the symptom

1 = Occasionally have it; the effect is not severe

2 = Occasionally have it; the effect is severe (it interferes with my life)

3 = Frequently have it; the effect is not severe

4 = Frequently have it; the effect is severe

Date_____

DIGESTIVE TRACT	HEAD	MOUTH/THROAT
Nausea or vomiting	Headaches	Chronic coughing
Diarrhea	Faintness	Gagging, need to clear throat
Constipation	Dizziness	Sore throat, hoarseness, loss of voice
Bloated feeling	Insomnia	
Belching or passing gas	Total: ___	Swollen/discolored tongue, gums, lips
Heartburn		Canker sores
Intestinal/stomach pain		
Total: ___		Total: ___
EARS	**HEART**	**NOSE**
Itchy ears	Irregular or skipped heartbeat	Stuffy nose
Earaches, ear infections		Sinus problems
Drainage from ear	Rapid or pounding heartbeat	Hay fever
Ringing in ears, hearing loss	Chest pain	Sneezing attacks
Total: ___	Total: ___	Excessive mucus formation
		Total: ___
EMOTIONS	**JOINTS/MUSCLES**	**SKIN**
Mood swings	Pain or aches in joints	Acne
Anxiety, fear, or nervousness	Arthritis	Hives, rashes, or dry skin
Anger, irritability, or aggressiveness	Stiffness or limitation of movement	Hair loss
	Pain or aches in muscles	Flushing or hot flashes
Depression	Feeling of weakness or tiredness	Excessive sweating
Total: ___		Total: ___
	Total: ___	

ENERGY/ACTIVITY	LUNGS	WEIGHT
Fatigue, sluggishness	Chest congestion	Binge eating/drinking
Apathy, lethargy	Asthma, bronchitis	Craving certain foods
Hyperactivity	Shortness of breath	Excessive weight
Restlessness	Difficulty breathing	Compulsive eating
Total: ___	Total: ___	Water retention
		Underweight
		Total: ___
EYES	**MIND**	**OTHER**
Watery or itchy eyes	Poor memory	Frequent illness
Swollen, reddened, or sticky eyelids	Confusion, poor comprehension	Frequent or urgent urination
Bags or dark circles under eyes	Poor concentration	Genital itch or discharge
Blurred or tunnel vision (does not include near- or farsightedness)	Poor physical coordination	Total: ___
Total: ___	Difficulty in making decisions	
	Stuttering or stammering	
	Slurred speech	
	Learning disabilities	
	Total: ___	

SCORING

OPTIMAL	MILD TOXICITY	MODERATE TOXICITY	SEVERE TOXICITY
< 10	10–50	50–100	> 100

The Eve Questionnaire

Eve was the original woman in the Bible. By most accounts—and judging from Adam's supposed fall from grace in her presence—she was seductive, confident, and sexual. I say, good for her! And therefore what better name to use for a questionnaire that aims to assess your sexual and pelvic health?

Once you know your starting number (from 0 to 70; lower is better), it's much easier to track your progress as you change your diet and implement lifestyle changes. Read through each question, and check off your response. (Many of the questions refer to symptoms with sex; if you're not sexually active, answer "never" or give your best guess.)

(Your response should reflect your sexual feelings and activity during the past ninety days.)

1. Do you lack energy?
   - ☐ Never
   - ☐ Some of the time
   - ☐ Quite often
   - ☐ Always

2. Do you find yourself making up excuses to avoid having sex?
   - ☐ Never
   - ☐ Some of the time
   - ☐ Quite often
   - ☐ Always

3. Do you find yourself sexually undesirable?
   - ☐ Never
   - ☐ Some of the time
   - ☐ Quite often
   - ☐ Always

4. Is the thought of sex distressing for you?
   - ☐ Never
   - ☐ Some of the time
   - ☐ Quite often
   - ☐ Always

5. Do you have discomfort during or after sex?
   - ☐ Never
   - ☐ Some of the time
   - ☐ Quite often
   - ☐ Always

6. Is vaginal or vulvar dryness troublesome?
  ☐ Never
  ☐ Some of the time
  ☐ Quite often
  ☐ Always

7. Would you consider yourself frustrated about your sex life?
  ☐ Never
  ☐ Some of the time
  ☐ Quite often
  ☐ Always

8. Do you find it very difficult to become aroused?
  ☐ Never
  ☐ Some of the time
  ☐ Quite often
  ☐ Always

9. Do you lose urine when you cough or sneeze?
  ☐ Never
  ☐ Some of the time
  ☐ Quite often
  ☐ Always

10. Do you use pads or panty liners due to urine leakage?
  ☐ Never
  ☐ Some of the time
  ☐ Quite often
  ☐ Always

SCORING

Review your answers. For every "Never," assign 0 points. For every "Some of the time," assign 3 points. For every "Quite often," assign 5 points. For every "Always," assign 7 points.

Record your total points: _____

Interpretation

If you scored between 0 and 10, you are doing extremely well. Your desire is healthy and intact, with normal vaginal and orgasmic function. But if you scored closer to 15, you may be experiencing some symptoms that could worsen over time, unless you take steps to improve them.

If you scored between 15 and 30, you are having a few arousal, vaginal health, and orgasmic functioning issues that are standing in the way of vibrant sexual health and vitality. Making lifestyle changes now will begin to lower your score.

If you scored between 31 and 50, your decreased interest in and enjoyment of sex may be due to a number of factors—vaginal pain problems, arousal issues, or urinary problems, among others. But these are all reversible with the right lifestyle changes.

If you scored above 50, your reduced interest in sex, your ability to become aroused, vaginal pain, or other sexual health issues are interfering with the quality of your sex life and pelvic health. These problems, though discouraging, can be improved or completely resolved with proper lifestyle actions, consistently followed.

If you answered number 5 positively at all, that is, you experience discomfort before or after sex, please follow up with your gynecologist or other qualified health care provider right away. It is important to rule out any other pathology, such as cervical, uterine, and/or ovarian cancer. Any symptoms that don't improve with my recommendations in this book should be evaluated by your doctor.

Positivity Self-Assessment Questionnaire

Although hot flashes grab most of the attention, mood swings are an equally common symptom not only among menopausal-age women but also among women in their thirties due to PMS and those in their forties as a result of perimenopause. Common complaints include irritability, depression, crying, anxiety, fatigue, sadness, tension, difficulty concentrating, and loss of interest in sex.

There's no need to despair, however—or to rely solely on antidepressants or tranquilizers, which are commonly too often prescribed. You can restore normal hormonal balance with natural methods you'll learn about throughout this book. When all your hormones are in sync, you're on your way to a happy, energized, and content life.

You'll notice that the questions below work with positive statements instead of negative inventories. This way, the questionnaire is not only diagnostic but also therapeutic: the more you say the statements to yourself silently or out loud, the better you feel about you.

Don't worry if you can't rate many (or any) of these statements with a high score (in this quiz, the higher the overall number, the better you are feeling). I had one client, Mandy, who was thirty-six at her first visit. She was struggling with moodiness, fatigue, and relationship issues. I gave her the Positivity Self-Assessment Questionnaire; she returned it with zeros all the way down! This showed me that she had a lot more than physiology to heal. And she did.

With this assessment, you can see how your moods respond to the natural approach in a quick and fun way. Record your feelings (as well as information about your menstrual flow and libido) at least weekly, according to the directions. You'll be surprised that in as soon as one month, you'll feel much better emotionally.

SCORING

In the boxes below, rate your moods according to these scores.

0 = Not at all

1 = Minimal

2 = Some

3 = Extremely

Also, on the dates you score your moods, note your menses too. Record one of the following letters under the date:

S = Spotting L = Light flow M = Average H = Heavy

For sexual activity, draw a smiley face ☺ under the date.

DATE ☺	I AM HAPPY AND JOYFUL.	I AM CONTENT.	I AM ENERGETIC.	I AM PRODUCTIVE.	I AM SOCIAL AND FRIENDLY.	I AM ALERT; MY MIND IS FOCUSED.	I FEEL GOOD ABOUT MY BODY.

Your Waist and Hip Measurements

One of the best indicators of your overall health is decidedly low-tech: putting a cloth measuring tape around your waist and hips to come up with your waist-to-hip ratio. It says a lot about your health. If you carry more weight around your middle than your hips, you may be at a higher risk of developing certain health conditions, including heart disease.

Prior to beginning my program, find your waist-to-hip ratio and record it and the date:

- Stand and place a tape measure around your bare middle, crossing your navel.
- Make sure the tape is horizontal and snug around your waist, but without compressing or digging into your skin.
- Breathe normally.
- Read the tape. Your waist measurement will be at the place on the tape where the zero end meets the slack end of the tape measure.
- For your hip measurement, stand with your feet together and place a tape measure around the widest part of your buttocks.
- Double-check. Repeat the measurements to make sure they are accurate. If different from the first time, measure a third time and take the average of the three numbers.

To calculate your waist-to-hip ratio, divide your waist measurement by your hip measurement (W ÷ H). For example, if you have a 27-inch waist measurement and a 38-inch hip measurement, your waist-to-hip ratio is .71. For women, a ratio of .80 or less is considered to be healthy or safe. (For men, a ratio of .90 is ideal.)

Just as your weight can fluctuate during the day, so can waist and hip measurements. For the most accurate comparisons, take your measurements at the same time each time. Repeat these measurements weekly or monthly.

Urine Testing

It is essential to make sure that your diet and lifestyle produce an alkaline effect on your body, and that you're in ketosis. Although it's not required, I highly recommend that you test your urine daily. You can do this through separate pH strips and ketone strips, available at your pharmacy. Or you can obtain dual-purpose (ketone and pH test strips) on my website at dranna.com/resources. Unlike blood tests, you can do a urine test at home and without the pain of a pinprick.

Test your urine first thing in the morning, and periodically throughout the day (especially to check pH).

To use the dual-purpose strips:

- As you urinate, pass the test end of the strip through your urine in midstream, or collect your urine in a clean, dry container or paper cup and dip the test strip in it.
- Blot excess drops of urine off the strip.
- Lay the strip flat on toilet paper or other absorbent paper.
- The test strip will change color to indicate whether or not ketones are being produced, and to show if your body is in an acidic or alkaline state.
- After 40 seconds, match to the ketone color chart.
- After 60 seconds, match to the pH color chart.
- Record your results on your Daily Tracker (see below).

Your urine pH goal should be in the 7 range in the morning. Don't worry if this takes you a while to achieve. Testing is a process of discovery. Some people will have lower pH to start with. That's okay as long as you are measuring it at the onset of this program; this is your baseline. You can track your pH from there in order to see what is happening over time and throughout the day. Patterns will emerge and show you how the food you eat and the way you live trigger changes in your pH.

The easiest way to monitor your progress to ketosis is through urine testing. A limitation of urine testing for ketones, however, is that urine tests measure the ketone acetoacetate, and less acetoacetate is spilled into the urine over time when we are consistently using fat for fuel or are keto-adapted. (Typically, this condition takes several weeks to develop.)

People ask me about blood testing for ketones. Yes, you can also test your blood for ketones (beta hydroxybutyrate is the ketone measured in blood) using a meter like the one diabetics use, along with special strips. The disadvantage to this method, however, is that some people don't like pricking themselves with a lancet. Also, the test strips are considerably more expensive, usually $2 to $5 per test. This can add up if you are testing often to track changes in ketone levels. Given all this, in my opinion urine testing is the best way to start; then use blood or even breath ketone testing for fine-tuning if needed.

Your Daily Tracker

The tracker I created below serves as a journal and accountability tool, where you'll record your feelings, weight, hours of sleep, ketones, pH, water intake, and other stats. It is important to keep track of these items, because they indicate your progress and help you stay the course. Don't worry about where you are starting, just think about where you are heading!

- Record your weight, waist measurement, and hip measurement at the beginning of each week.
- Start off each day by writing down what you are grateful for.
- Set your intentions for the day—in other words, what you want to accomplish, enjoy, experience, or improve in your life.
- Choose a "cheer word." This is a word that when you say or think of it it brings a smile to your face. Maybe it is a word like "jiggle," or the name of your child, love, or pet, or even the word "smile." Say this word many times throughout the day to bring a smile to your face, instead of a "resting witch face."
- Write down what or whom you have connected with this day.
- Write what oxytocin activity you did or plan to do. Did you laugh, play, share intimacy, or enjoy friendships, for example? These positive activities bring more oxytocin into our lives, which can be so fruitful.

- Next is a brief positivity self-assessment questionnaire, which I shared earlier. Where an item is marked with a double asterisk (**), fill in the daily blanks with one of the following scores:

  0 = Not at all
  1 = Slightly
  2 = More often
  3 = Absolutely

For example, for "body love," say "I love my body" and assess how that statement makes you feel. Hopefully you are answering with an "absolutely" and recording a 3. If you're not yet, take heart—you will be soon.

Next are vital signs, because they will give you more clues as to how your body is responding to what you are doing.

- Recording your weight daily at the start is very helpful because if you note a sudden bump up, it may signal a food sensitivity, stressful day, or hormonal issue, all of which can provide more clues.
- Record your hours of sleep from the night before.
- Record your urine pH and ketones throughout the day.
- Record your water intake.
- Check if you added an alkalinizer to your diet, like Mighty Maca Plus (MM), baking soda (B), or apple cider vinegar (ACV).
- Check if you've had that all-important bowel movement each day.
- List what physical activity you enjoyed.
- Note why today was great! Keep your focus on the positives.

See dranna.com/resources for a helpful video that walks you through this tracker.

Week Starting_____

Height _____ Weight _____ Waist _____ Hips_____

	MONDAY	TUESDAY	WEDNESDAY	THURSDAY	FRIDAY	SATURDAY	SUNDAY
Intentions:							
Grateful for:							
Cheer word:							
Connected with:							
Oxytocin activity:							
**Joyful							
**Content							
**Energetic							
**Productive							
**Friendly							
**Focused							
**Body love							
Weight:							
Hours of sleep:							
pH:							
Ketones:							
Water intake:							
MM/B/ACV:							
Bowel movement:							
Physical activity today:							
Why today was great:							

Laboratory Testing

You've probably done it lots of times in your life: rolled up your sleeve and given a sample of blood, or urinated in a cup at your doctor's office. A week or two later, you receive a lab report with a long list of measurements, ranges, and numbers. The whole process can seem a little confusing, but all that information helps your doctor paint a picture of your overall health. So your lab results are essentially a checkup on how your organs are operating, as well as an assessment of your risk for cardiovascular disease, diabetes, and other conditions. If you're basically healthy, you can probably have lab work done every two to three years. But if you have coronary artery disease, diabetes, or risk factors for them, you should probably have lab tests done more often.

My patients and participants in my online menopause program always ask me about lab testing. In my experience, time, money, and worry can be saved by performing the self-tests in this chapter regularly. These provide a guide to what you need to know about your midlife health and hormones. Lab testing is completely optional and not a part of this program.

That said, if you are interested in optional lab testing, there are four key and inexpensive blood tests that I do think are worthwhile and cost-effective. They give you critical information that I believe every adult should know and follow periodically. Why these four? From an economical and informational standpoint, these tests clue you in to your immune resilience, inflammation status, blood sugar control, and hormonal status—basically a comprehensive overview of what is happening in your body. They also enable us to measure improvement as you work to optimize these values. (These four tests typically cost under $125 total; see dranna.com/resources page.)

> **25-hydroxy vitamin D.** This blood test monitors vitamin D levels in your body and can determine if levels are too high or low. It is an important indicator of bone weakness or strength, immunity, mood, and more. Vitamin D and your vital hormone progesterone work together to support T cell immunity and sex hormone functions. Higher vitamin D levels are associated with reduced cancer

risk (including breast cancer), better mood, better memory, brain health, and strong bones. A normal reading is 30–80 ng/mL; optimal is 50–100 ng/mL.

hsC-reactive protein test (also known as cardio-CRP and highly sensitive CRP). This blood test is a sensitive marker of inflammation and is used to help diagnose infection, cancer, and immune system disorders such as lupus and arthritis, as well as to help screen for heart disease. Normal CRP levels are below 3.0 mg/dL; optimal levels are below 1.0 mg/dL.

Hemoglobin A1c. This blood test shows your average level of blood sugar control over the past two to three months. People who have diabetes need this test regularly to check their progression or improvement of disease. We can use it to show that our nutrition and lifestyle choices are working. While the hemoglobin A1c (HbA1c) test is used to diagnose diabetes when it is 6.5 percent or higher, much research has shown that every 0.1 percentage point above 5.3 percent significantly increases your risk for Alzheimer's disease, brain shrinkage, and cancer. HbA1c levels between 5.7 and 6.4 percent mean pre-diabetes. The normal range is between 4 and 5.6 percent; optimal is under 5.3 percent. Everyone should know their number and get it optimal.

DHEA-sulfate. This blood test measures the amount of DHEA-sulfate in the blood. DHEA-sulfate is a biomarker of aging and a way to assess the functioning of the adrenal glands and the effectiveness of communication along the body's hypothalamic-pituitary-adrenal (HPA) axis. It is also a precursor hormone to estrogen and testosterone.

Low levels are associated with insulin resistance, poor memory, immune disease, and atherosclerosis. Optimal DHEA-S levels are associated with protection against cardiovascular disease and cancer, decreased risk of osteoporosis, healthier bones and immune system, better memory, better cognition, and better sexual function.

Typical normal ranges for women are:*

Ages 30 to 39: 45 to 270 μg/dL or 1.22 to 7.29 μmol/L

Ages 40 to 49: 32 to 240 μg/dL or 0.86 to 6.48 μmol/L

Ages 50 to 59: 26 to 200 μg/dL or 0.70 to 5.40 μmol/L

Ages 60 to 69: 13 to 130 μg/dL or 0.35 to 3.51 μmol/L

Ages 69 and older: 17 to 90 μg/dL or 0.46 to 2.43 μmol/L

Other Lab Tests Worth Considering

The four tests discussed above are really important in determining your hormonal and overall health. This chart shows other common and specialty tests that your doctor may want to order. All are good and helpful, and I regularly use them in my private practice.

TEST	WHAT IT TESTS	METHOD
Comprehensive metabolic and hormone panel	Complete blood count (CBC), complete metabolic panel, cortisol, DHEA-sulfate (if not done separately), estrogen, progesterone, testosterone, hemoglobin A1c, C-reactive protein, blood lipids, red blood cell magnesium, vitamin D, and thyroid hormones (free T4, free T3, and thyroid antibodies, among others). Additional tests, depending on individual needs, might include a ferritin and iron panel.	Blood test

---

* Optimal ranges are 100–250 μg/dL in women over 40.

Comprehensive stool analysis (such as GI Effects or GI-Map)	This test gives a comprehensive look at the overall health of the gastrointestinal tract. It can reveal important clinical information about common symptoms such as gas, bloating, indigestion, abdominal pain, diarrhea, constipation, and the possible presence of parasites, yeast, and small intestinal bacterial overgrowth known as SIBO.	Stool sample
Gluten-associated cross-reactive foods and food sensitivity (Array 4) and epithelial permeability test (Array 2) from Cyrex Labs	Array 4 is my favorite panel for gluten sensitivity testing. This test measures your body's immune response to various gluten-containing foods. Two antibodies are usually measured: IgA and IgG. Array 2 measures certain proteins and can be an earlier and less expensive indicator of disease and leaky gut, reasons for chronic fatigue syndrome, and immune disease.	Blood test
Food sensitivity test from Cell Science Systems	This is a comprehensive test I have used to uncover which foods and other substances might be triggering inflammation and related issues such as digestive problems, metabolic disorders, and chronic inflammatory symptoms such as fatigue, migraines, eczema, autoimmune disorders, and joint pain. This test measures reactions to more than 450 substances (food, chemical, and environmental substances).	Blood test

Adrenal stress index	This test gives a more comprehensive understanding of adrenal hormone balance by assessing cortisol and DHEA throughout the day. It is an ideal evaluation for those under chronic stress with known or suspected endocrine abnormalities. It tests for six different hormones and immune markers that may be affected by chronic stress and stress-related conditions.	Saliva test
23andMe Ancestry and Health	This test provides genetic health risk reports, wellness reports (sleep, weight, lactose intolerance, and so forth), carrier status for a variety of conditions, including late-onset Alzheimer's disease, celiac disease, Parkinson's disease, and various genetic-related disorders. This health data can then be evaluated by a knowledgeable health care provider for guidance.	Saliva test
Urinary testing for hormones and nutrition from Precision Analytics or Genova	This test identifies hormones and their metabolites over a full 24-hour period. Especially important if there is history of breast cancer or you are on HRT.	At-home urine testing

Take these self-discovery assessments diligently—and discuss these lab tests with your physician. The information you'll gain will help you on your journey of mastering your midlife hormones and claiming optimal health for the rest of your life.

Chapter 3

What Is the Hormone Fix?

So what exactly is the Hormone Fix? What does it involve?

The Hormone Fix is a novel breakthrough diet with enhanced lifestyle strategies that is designed to balance your hormones. As an ob-gyn, I'd love to tell you that this involves tweaking those familiar reproductive hormones—progesterone, estrogen, testosterone, and DHEA—but it's not, at least not directly. The Hormone Fix focuses on mastering three control hormones: insulin, cortisol, and oxytocin. When those are in balance, your other hormones turn into a sweet, beautiful hormonal symphony.

Central to making this happen is a combination of a modified ketogenic diet and an alkaline diet, or what I call my Keto-Green Diet. What you eat is 25 percent of the whole picture. Lifestyle changes make up the other 75 percent of the Hormone Fix program.

Historically, when I put women on a ketogenic diet—a diet that is high in good fats, adequate in protein, and very low in carbohydrates—because I believed it would help them lose weight rapidly, improve energy, and boost memory, they'd invariably complain about feeling miserable and cranky. I knew exactly what they were talking about. I felt the same way on a keto diet—I call it going "keto crazy." And that just wouldn't do. However, I was forty-eight at the time, with my menopausal hormone imbalance and stressful life situations, and I was gaining weight again, experiencing memory issues and brain fog, so I needed a better solution and I needed it fast!

I dug into the medical research. I found an obscure journal article published in 1924 in the *Biochemical Journal* from the Biochemical Laboratory in Cambridge, England. It pointed out that making a ketogenic diet more alkaline could be very beneficial and therapeutic. This information gave me an aha moment. What if I put more alkalinizing foods such as greens and other veggies into my version of the ketogenic diet? After all, when you stay in ketosis (a fat-burning state) too long—this is especially true for women—your body becomes acidic, creating chronic inflammation that forces your body to hold on to its fat stores. I've seen this play out numerous times among my female patients.

I decided to be my own guinea pig. I checked my urine repeatedly with strips that measured ketones (signs of fat-burning) and pH (a measure of urine [not blood] acidity and alkalinity). As it turned out, I was persistently acidic, brought on by strict low-carb eating. No wonder I felt irritable.

My diet clearly needed a major alkaline boost. More on this later, but in brief, too many acidic foods in your diet can upset hormone balance, hurt your immune system, inhibit digestion, increase metabolic syndrome, cause osteoporosis, and contribute to premature aging, not to mention, make you feel nuts!

I refined the diet to include more alkaline vegetables that support hormone balance (especially green veggies, hence the name Keto-Green Diet), along with dietary strategies to maintain a fat-burning state initiated by ketogenic nutrition. Very quickly I felt better. I stayed in a fat-burning mode longer, without any unpleasant side effects. I lost my extra weight and kept it off. I felt energized. The combination of keto and alkaline eating made all the difference.

I then turned on eight of my friends and patients—my first test panel!—to my Keto-Green idea. I created for them a diet and lifestyle plan that was both ketogenic and alkalinizing. I asked them to follow it for eight weeks and measure their ketones, pH, weight loss, and attitudes. Seriously, there's no sense in looking good if you're not feeling good!

Their results were amazing! They all lost pounds rapidly. They were generally not hungry and had no cravings. Each of them saw their hemoglobin A1c drop (this is a general measure of how well blood sugar is controlled). Even their C-reactive protein (CRP) fell, indicating that there was less health-damaging inflammation going on in their bodies. Also, to a woman, they eliminated their annoying menopause symptoms such as hot flashes . . . all without going crazy.

Pretty soon I put more and more clients on the keto-alkaline diet, now christened my Keto-Green Diet. I observed and recorded their results, and eventually connected the dots, realizing that there is a lot more to this than diet alone. Lifestyle, from sleep habits to stress management, also makes a huge impact in the quality of our lives and relationships—which is what women really want upgraded at this point in their lives.

All of my experience and research had now come full circle. I discovered that the best way to lose weight and ensure optimal health is to combine an alkaline diet and lifestyle changes, along with getting into ketosis.

Seemingly like magic—but very much based on science—the Keto-Green Diet works wonders for all women, including those in the tenacious stages of fluctuating hormones associated with perimenopause, menopause, or postmenopause. No one else had addressed any of this in the medical or nutritional communities. No one had put the pieces together before. But after all my work and observations, and seeing the results with my own eyes, I knew I had the answers for millions of women, including you.

I was encouraged and inspired when I realized that this would work for women of all ages, but especially for those in the midst of or going through menopause. In this population of women, doctors are seeing an increase in cardiovascular disease, cancer, premature aging, and Alzheimer's disease. The current medical approach medicalizes and stigmatizes menopause. I prefer to first take a holistic approach whenever possible. With this we could reduce the number of expensive medications and invasive procedures that may cause serious side effects and even harm.

The bottom line is that proponents of ketogenesis got it partly right by utilizing ketones as fuel. So did alkaline-diet folks by recognizing how crucial staying alkaline becomes to staying lean, sane, and healthy.

So combine the two and then add the lifestyle component, and *bam*— you've got a really powerful plan that uniquely balances female hormones and results in rapid energy, mental clarity, reduced hot flashes, and many other incredible changes. It is exactly what you need to get slim, feel sexy, and be in control once again.

The Role of Ketosis in the Hormone Fix

So how does this all work?

The word "ketogenic" means "ketone-producing," a reference to the splitting of fat molecules into ketones, which, like sugars, can be converted into energy. Your cells then switch over from burning sugar to burning fat. When this happens, you are in ketosis. Your body is using fat as its primary fuel source in the absence of carbs.

A ketogenic diet is traditionally very high in fat and very low in carbohydrates, with adequate amounts of protein. As a result, foods such as breads, cereals, pasta, rice, and potatoes are essentially eliminated from this diet. Although keto diets typically include dairy, I eliminate most dairy foods on the 10-Day Keto-Green Quick Start Detox due to their carbohydrate content and the fact that they can trigger food sensitivities in some people, as well as hormone disruptions.

Ketogenic nutrition is based on thousands of years of history. If you go back in time, way before twenty-four-hour supermarkets, restaurants, and refrigerators, even before humans figured out how to farm, our ancestors were eating meats they hunted and vegetables they gathered. Their meals were low-carb and included plenty of animal protein and lots of fat. They were the first keto dieters. In general, men would eat more of the meats and fats than women, because they needed more of those nutrients for energy to hunt and protect the tribe.

You might be wondering what the difference is between a strictly ketogenic diet and a paleo diet, since both are tied to ancestral nutrition. Paleo eaters base their diet on what our Paleolithic ancestors would have eaten, and they restrict grains, dairy, legumes, processed foods, and alcohol. They typically have a higher carbohydrate intake and don't worry about getting into ketosis. The major difference is that a keto diet is typically higher in healthy fats and lower in carbohydrates than a paleo plan. It also does not villainize any specific food group. You can be paleo and follow a ketogenic plan. My Keto-Green plan pulls in the best of both, for hormone-balancing, while emphasizing alkalinizing foods as well as intermittent fasting and lifestyle factors.

Worth noting too is that our ancestors got up with the sun and walked an average of ten miles every day, staking out new settlement possibilities, exploring uncharted territories, or searching for food. At night, they went to bed just after dark. Depending on the time of year, they probably got eight to ten hours of sleep. This ancient, nomadic lifestyle meant that they often endured extended periods of time without eating.

Today we call this "intermittent fasting," and it is a key component in achieving ketosis. Essentially, in my Keto-Green plan, it involves going thirteen to fifteen hours without food between dinner and breakfast the next day. Some of the benefits of intermittent fasting are that it accelerates fat-burning, allows the food you've eaten to completely digest and your gut to rest, and supports a robust population of healthy gut bacteria, which is essential for hormones and weight control. You'll learn how to apply intermittent fasting in Chapter 4.

There is evidence in fossil records that our ancient ancestors lived well into old age—if they survived the perilous period of infancy to age fifteen, when young people died off from disease, injuries, and accidents. Their natural diets, along with daily periods of not eating, probably helped by supporting their immune system.

In more modern times, anthropologists have watched native tribes develop obesity and diabetes in just a few generations after being introduced to complex carbohydrates such as wheat and rice. Why is this? We have the same genes as our ancient ancestors—genes that are adapted to a natural diet in which food was hunted, fished, or gathered. But today we eat from a vastly different food supply with processed foods full of refined sugars, salt, unhealthy fats, and questionable additives and preservatives, resulting in a society riddled with obesity, cancer, autism in children, and other diseases. We are exposed daily to toxins and unnatural substances in our foods to the detriment of our health and the health of our children—a situation that angers me as a doctor, scientist, and mom. Our genes—which are survivor genes (not fat genes)—just can't handle modern diets.

I recall many times when moms tearfully brought their young teen daughters to see me. After starting their periods, these girls began gaining weight, along with getting terrible acne and suffering from cramps and moodiness. They worried that they were destined to be "fat" and "ugly." What I told these beautiful young women was that they don't have "fat" genes, but they do have Pocahontas genes or Amazonian genes. That gives them a more positive image of themselves. I told them they are designed to thrive and survive in harsh conditions. As long as they get back to nature and eat foods they can pick, peel, fish, hunt, milk, and grow versus the processed and packaged foods, they can stay naturally thin and fit. It's basically the same message I give to older women going through menopause and beyond. We need to honor our design with natural food and natural living through our various life stages.

One of the keys to doing so is the ketogenic diet. This diet strictly restricts carbohydrates, which are energy foods, including starchy carbs such as potatoes, as well as fruit and sugary processed carbs. For most of our lives, we use glucose from carbs to fuel our bodies. But come midlife, the body cannot metabolize a lot of carbs—or fats, for that matter—as well as it used to, due to shifting hormones, enzymes, and gut bacteria. We become metabolically stalled and very good energy conservers, which causes weight gain. We truly just don't need as many carbs.

When we eat carbs the digestive system dismantles them into glucose, which is sugar. The pancreas releases insulin to drive that sugar into muscle cells, liver cells, and fat cells to be used as energy. We certainly need energy, but most of us spend our days living indoors in relative ease. So after all this energy goes unused by our muscles, insulin drives that extra blood sugar into our fat stores "just in case" we need it later. Insulin is a fat storage hormone, and even more of it is cranked out when we eat a lot of carbs, snack throughout the day, and eat late at night.

Because most of us never need that stored fat later, those fat deposits build up day after day, week after week, month after month, and year after year. If you continue to eat a high-carb diet (and you have lots of insulin in your system), your body gets stuck in that fat storage mode. That means more pounds, more cellulite, and more belly fat—and a higher risk of cancer, heart disease, dementia, and poor quality of life. These health bombs certainly aren't what we've worked so hard for, and for so long!

Keto eating and getting into ketosis defuses these bombs—and helps restore hormone balance and health. Here's what you gain from getting your body into ketosis, especially the Keto-Green way.

Ketosis Prevents Insulin Resistance

Beyond the visible weight gain from eating too many carbs, there is the less visible: a dangerous, insidious condition called insulin resistance. Insulin resistance occurs when your body can't take proper command of insulin, which is required to usher glucose into cells for energy. As a result, the pancreas reacts by churning out more insulin, so blood levels of the hormone begin to rise. Over time, the cells simply can't keep up. They stop responding to the insulin and become insulin resistant. Insulin resistance also puts you on the road to full-blown type 2 diabetes.

To better understand this, think of insulin like a key that unlocks the cell doors to let glucose in. If the key and lock on the door are new and well oiled, the key turns readily without a lot of force and the lock opens smoothly. Insulin resistance, on the other hand, is like an old rusty lock on that door. The key won't turn, the lock doesn't work, the doorknob can't turn, and insulin is shut out. You are then insulin resistant.

A ketogenic diet prevents and reverses insulin resistance. In fact, it makes you insulin sensitive, so you don't have to worry as much about high blood sugar, weight gain, and various menopausal symptoms—especially hot flashes (one cause of which is insulin resistance).

I've seen this happen in client after client. Stacy is a great example. At age fifty-three she was struggling with declining health, fatigue, and "hormone hell" (as she put it), and had a strong family history of diabetes, which affected both parents and all her siblings. Being her own best advocate, she tested her hemoglobin A1c level and it was 5.6 percent, meaning borderline pre-diabetic. While it is true that the normal range for HbA1c is between 4 and 5.6 percent, levels between 5.7 and 6.4 percent indicate you are pre-diabetic—that is, you have a higher chance of or are on your way to becoming a diabetic. And every 0.1 percentage point increase above 5.3 percent significantly increases the risk of diabetes, Alzheimer's, dementia, cardiovascular disease, and more. She wasn't willing to wait for a diagnosis to do something about it. After following the Hormone Fix, Stacy reduced her HbA1c to 5.0 percent in a year, reducing her risk of diabetes and improving her overall health greatly. Now she is active on her farm, riding horses and "tinkering away," as she says, because she has the energy to do so.

Ketosis Optimizes Your Blood Sugar

Eating ketogenically is especially helpful for people with type 2 diabetes, but it is beneficial to almost everyone. This is because a keto diet optimizes blood sugar and insulin levels. Scientific studies among people with type 2 diabetes have found such dramatic glucose improvements that patients were able to discontinue or reduce their diabetes medications—as my father did when he was seventy-nine.

So if you want to regulate insulin and blood sugar and get your body out of a fat-storing mode, you need a scarcity of carbohydrates. With fewer carbs, your body goes looking for other energy sources. After about three days without carbs, most of the insulin retreats from your system, and your body will go into ketosis and start burning fat.

Ketosis Tames Your Appetite

A ketogenic diet also curbs your appetite and stops your cravings. Eating fat and protein stabilizes hormones that control your appetite and makes you feel fuller. One of those hormones is leptin. Secreted by fat cells, leptin is nicknamed the "satiety hormone" because it sends a message to your brain that you are full and don't need to eat any more.

But if your body gets into a fat-storing mode, due mostly to snacking or eating too many carbs, more leptin is produced. When that happens, the body eventually stops hearing the hormonal messages telling it to stop eating. It is like the begging dog at the dinner table whom you tune out while you just keep eating your meal, not paying any attention (you know what I mean). This is termed "leptin resistance." Eating ketogenically prevents leptin resistance—and therefore reduces cravings. I used to have intense food cravings that made me think of food all the time, but after going more keto, I was liberated from them, and I can't wait for you to experience this too.

Ketosis Prevents Disease

The ketogenic diet is also effective in certain medical situations. It is a treatment modality used today for people with seizure disorders, such as epilepsy, because ketones cross the blood-brain barrier and make for good brain fuel.

Keto diets have also been used in the treatment of cancer. When a person adopts a ketogenic diet, several anti-cancer changes occur. Ketone levels increase, and glucose levels decrease. Cancer cells—which like to gobble up glucose—are thus starved, so they tend to self-destruct. Good news for women: studies show that a ketogenic state, combined with intermittent fasting, can lower your risk of developing breast cancer.

Ketosis Improves Memory

The brain requires estrogen to metabolize glucose, the primary brain fuel, as well as support the health of our mitochondria (energy factories within each cell). But when estrogen falls off, our brains get deprived of fuel. This is a reason we experience "brain fog" and are at risk for age-related brain disorders like Alzheimer's disease. Fortunately, ketones can cross the blood-brain barrier and become the ideal brain fuel for improving memory and clarity.

The Downside of Keto Eating Without the Green

As you can see, there are many great reasons to get started on a ketogenic diet, but I wouldn't be doing my duty as a doctor if I didn't warn you about a few issues.

Keto Flu

Many people on this type of diet experience what's called the "keto flu," as their body gets used to burning ketones for fuel instead of glucose. The most common symptoms are headache and fatigue, but some people also experience nausea, upset stomach, and brain fog.

Keto flu usually lasts only a few days, but in rare cases it can last up to two weeks. If you can get past the keto flu, you'll experience a few weeks of magic: more mental clarity and energy with less hunger. You may also drop a dress size or two, watch your skin improve, and see mysterious aches and pains simply disappear.

I know what you're thinking: "This sounds wonderful! I'm going to stay on a ketogenic diet the rest of my life!" But then all of a sudden you feel terrible, like the keto flu, only worse, thanks to . . .

Keto Craziness

A ketogenic diet that's very carb restrictive can, at least temporarily, wreak havoc on your mental state by messing with brain chemicals that help stabilize mood. I call this going "keto crazy." I've experienced this myself, and all I can say is that it turned me into a witch! I've heard this complaint from my premenopausal patients too.

There's an entire cascade of hormonal events that can throw you into keto craziness as you get older. You see, when you're younger, your body makes a lot of the hormone progesterone, a neuroprotective hormone that is vital to brain health. I call it the "calm, cool, collected hormone." With progesterone in ample supply, your body can better tolerate a keto diet.

Progesterone increases an important brain chemical known as brain-derived neurotrophic factor (BDNF). It preserves the brain's ability to grow and change through the years in response to new challenges, and to resist depression, memory loss, brain shrinkage, and other problems. Progesterone also prevents cell death in brain cells, protects the sheaths around nerves, and reduces the anxiety-provoking effects of glutamate, another type of brain chemical.

The challenge after your thirties is that progesterone begins to decline, and with it, the ability to fully protect your brain and nerves. Low progesterone also causes levels of gamma-aminobutyric acid (GABA) to fall off. GABA is an amino acid and one of the brain's chief calming neurotransmitters. When you're low on GABA, you tend to become more anxious, depressed, and sleep deprived—all of which lead to keto craziness if you go on a 100 percent keto diet without the green (alkaline) factor.

Increased Toxicity

Every day, we ingest and are exposed to thousands of chemicals from processed foods, heavy metals, pesticides, personal care products, and prescription drugs. To guard your health against these worrisome toxins, the body likes to store them in fat tissue. Think of that tissue like storage units you rent to stash your extra stuff. The more stuff you accumulate, the more space you need for storage. Your body works the same way. It hangs on to fat so there is enough storage space for toxins. But after you get into ketosis and start breaking down that fat, that toxic payload is discharged into your system.

When toxins hit your system, free radicals are generated. These are unstable atoms or molecules that contain one or more unpaired electrons in their outer orbit. Free radicals attempt to become stable by "stealing" electrons from cell membranes.

Like the borders in your garden that keep weeds from invading your plants, cell membranes protect cells from free radical invasion. If cell membranes are penetrated by these molecular invaders, more free radicals—like fast-growing weeds—are generated. A chain reaction is set into motion that eventually results in cellular damage and disease. In the short term, free radical attacks can make you feel inflamed and foggy-brained; in the longer term, they can cause memory loss, heart disease, stroke, Parkinson's disease, and many degenerative diseases.

Increased Acidity

A ketogenic diet can also make your system more acidic than usual if you are eating more acidic foods, like meat and cheese, and forgoing certain necessary alkalinizing vegetables (more on this below). Frankly, this is not ideal in the long term for women, especially menopausal women. It's healthier for your body to be in an alkaline state, in which you will feel energized and healthy.

IS A STRICT AND STRAIGHT KETO DIET RIGHT FOR EVERYONE?

My answer is no. You should not follow a 100 percent keto diet without physician guidance if you:

- Have liver or kidney disease
- Have suffered a recent heart attack
- Are a type 2 diabetic taking oral medications for your condition
- Have type 1 diabetes
- Have severe hypoglycemia
- Are pregnant or nursing
- Have been diagnosed with symptomatic gallstones
- Have the APOE4 gene (a gene commonly associated with late-onset Alzheimer's disease)

The Role of Alkalinity in the Hormone Fix

In simple terms, an alkaline diet is a way of eating that emphasizes non-acidifying foods over acidifying ones. You base your food choices around those that lower the acid levels in your body. It is a versatile diet that suits all of us.

As with keto eating, data about our early human ancestors suggests that once upon a time humans consumed mostly an alkaline diet—so in truth our ancestors were eating a Keto-Green Diet!

A study published in *The American Journal of Clinical Nutrition* in 2003 analyzed 159 hypothetical pre-agricultural diets (since we don't know for sure exactly what our ancestors ate ten thousand years ago). It found that 87 percent of these diets were "net base producing"—which means they were eating an alkaline diet, not an acidic one.

By contrast, the average Western diet has been shown to be "net acid producing." We already know that this sort of diet has created an obesity epidemic and is causing health issues such as cancer, heart disease, and a range of neurological disorders. Now it is becoming clearer that an alkaline diet may help prevent many of these illnesses. One reason is that it is better matched to our genetic makeup and supports healthy and diverse gut microbiota.

To understand alkalinity, let's flash back to high school chemistry, where you'll probably remember studying pH and acids versus bases (alkaline substances). If you can't recall, or would rather not go back mentally, let me provide a brief refresher course.

We measure pH on a scale ranging from 0 to 14, with 0 at the acid end, 14 at the alkaline end, and 7 being neutral (pH stands for "power of hydrogen"; it measures the total hydrogen ion concentration in a solution). The ocean has a pH of about 8.1. Your pool? An optimal pH for a pool is 7.4, which mirrors the pH of the human eyes, as well as the pH of our mucous membranes.

The human body works hard around the clock to maintain a slightly alkaline pH level in the blood, and to do so, it must clear out any excess of acid. Your body has a precise mechanism for maintaining its blood acid-base balance, and the mechanism ensures that the pH of blood doesn't shift much at all. It is tightly controlled by the kidneys and lungs to stay at around 7.4, with a very tight range from 7.35 to 7.45. This is critical for human life, because even a small variation in blood pH is life-threatening. This tight regulation declines with age, and there can be an increase in metabolic acidosis because most modern diets are acidic. That's another reason why eating alkaline is even more important as we age.

While the blood pH stays in a very small range, the rest of your body varies in pH level. Your stomach, for example, is very acidic, typically maintaining a pH of less than 3.0 so that it can fully break down the food you eat and kill ingested pathogens. The pH of your vagina is 3.8–4.4, which is protective and kills off unwanted bacteria, but this pH increases as we age. The skin has a pH below 5. By contrast, the pH of the intestines and pancreas is 8.0. Most cells work best when they are on the al-kaline side. The pH of urine, however, fluctuates and serves as a window on what is happening at the cellular and hormonal level. Ideally, it is good to see the pH of urine at 7, on average. After intense exercise, we expect it to be more acidic; after a relaxing day in nature, it will likely be more alkaline.

The pH of every system in the body is fine-tuned to its function. Think about it this way: the acidic systems, as a rule, protect and are a first line of defense against pathogens for your body. The alkaline systems nourish, restore, and repair. And the food you eat and the lifestyle you live impact that balance.

Which Foods Are Acidic and Which Are Alkaline

When you're in doubt about what's acidic and what's alkaline, ask yourself two simple questions: Does this food grow from the ground or on a tree? If so, it is probably alkaline, but not always. The other question is whether the food is a flesh food from an animal. Animal flesh foods such as meats are acidic. So are processed foods, especially those with sugar, artificial sweeteners, salt, and other added ingredients. In Appendix A you'll find a detailed list of alkaline foods, organized according to their carb content. But here's a chart that illustrates what I mean conceptually:

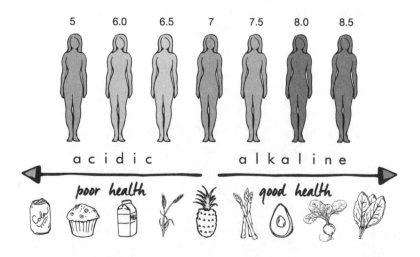

Some foods have a different pH outside the body than they do inside the body, however. Lemons are a good example. Outside the body, they are an acidic fruit with a pH of 2, but they have an alkalinizing effect inside the body. In fact, lemons confer great alkalinizing effects and are healthful in many ways.

In general, fruits, vegetables, certain vegetable oils, herbs and spices, and nuts and seeds are the most alkaline, due to their nutrient content. Meat, poultry, dairy, sugar, processed foods, caffeine, alcohol, and so forth are the most acidic. Of course, there are some outliers: grains, which grow from the ground, are slightly acidic. And some carbs, such as potatoes and sweet potatoes, are alkaline. As mentioned, you have to be careful about eating a lot of carbs, even the alkaline choices, because doing so can prevent your hormones from getting back in balance and your body from going into ketosis. The diet plans I provide in this book will guide you.

As I have alluded to earlier, staying alkaline is not only about food. There is also a huge lifestyle component that is key.

Recently, a friend of mine celebrated one evening with a meal of largely acidic foods—cocktails, beef, and a chocolate dessert. The next morning she tested her urine. To her surprise, she was quite alkaline. Why? Well, the fun, laughter, and love she shared with her friends ignited production of two feel-good hormones—oxytocin and dopamine—and decreased her stress hormone, cortisol. The result: more alkalinity. In other words, food is only part of the picture!

In fact, only about 25 to 50 percent of becoming alkaline is dietary; the other 50 to 75 percent is influenced by lifestyle factors. These factors include your level of hydration, how much you sleep and exercise, how positive you are (and, conversely, how stressed you are), how often you have bowel movements, and how much you are in touch with nature (getting natural light, walking barefoot, and so forth). This is fascinating, and you'll learn more about it in Part Three.

The Benefits of Becoming More Alkaline

In general, an alkaline diet prevents acidosis, which is at the root of many diseases. If your diet (and lifestyle) is too acidic—say, you're a habitual diet cola drinker—your body's overall pH load becomes overly acidic and can result in something called chronic low-grade acidosis. This indicates extreme acidity in your body. With it, a lot of your mineral levels, such as magnesium, calcium, and potassium, are likely to be low. This is where negative impacts to your health hit hard.

Alkalinity Impacts Bone Health

If your diet doesn't supply enough alkaline minerals or they become depleted from a continued acidic eating pattern and lifestyle over time, your body is forced to pull alkalinizing mineral buffers (calcium and magnesium) from its primary mineral storage reserves—your skeleton—in order to provide vital minerals throughout your system to maintain blood pH balance. Over time, this robbing of key buffering minerals can demineralize and weaken your bones. Indeed, in a study published in 2005 in *The Journal of Clinical Endocrinology & Metabolism*, both pre- and postmenopausal women and older men eating an acid-forming diet were found to have lower bone mineral density in the spine and hip. Bone mineral density is a measurement of the level of minerals in the bones, which indicates how dense and strong they are.

But if you eat more alkaline foods, particularly vegetables, your bone density increases, protecting you from bone-crippling osteoporosis. Many studies have been done supporting this conclusion. For example, a 2011 study from researchers in Seoul, Korea, studied postmenopausal Korean women with osteoporosis (and age-matched controls) and found that vegetables were an important source of calcium, other minerals, and vitamins that strengthened bone. Postmenopausal women who ate a vegetable-rich diet were able to boost their bone mineral density. In contrast, other studies have shown that diets high in dairy foods actually cause a reduction in bone mineral density.

Alkalinity Helps Your Heart

Heart disease is another health issue related to a high-acid diet. Just as acid rain eats away at stone, metal, and paint—almost any material exposed to the weather for a long period of time—acidosis irritates and inflames bodily tissue. The acids wear away the cell membranes, including the interiors of blood vessels and the very fabric of the heart. This ongoing process of erosion weakens the heart and vessels to the point where they are very susceptible to breakdown. Some studies show that as acidosis rises, there is a rise in homocysteine, an amino acid normally present in blood. However, at high levels, homocysteine is a risk factor for numerous cardiovascular diseases, including atherosclerosis, or clogging of the arteries, in which these blood vessels become less elastic and blood flow is impaired. I compare blood flow to traffic. When highways are congested, vehicles move slowly. Likewise, when arteries are clogged, blood moves sluggishly. The extra effort required to pump blood also boosts blood pressure, which is not a good thing.

Acidosis increases the production of the stress hormone cortisol—another risk factor for heart disease. (More on cortisol in Chapters 1 and 8.) Proof of this was reported in 2008 in the *British Journal of Nutrition*. Japanese women with acidosis caused by diet were shown to have higher systolic and diastolic blood pressure, putting them at risk for heart problems. Alkaline diets, on the other hand, reduce and control levels of cortisol. So when you switch to an alkaline diet and lifestyle, you prevent the dire consequences of acidosis.

Alkalinity Improves Fat-Burning

An alkaline diet assists the body in burning fat. First, as I mentioned, alkalinity (along with a low-carb diet) decreases levels of cortisol. Second, an alkaline diet helps you work out more intensely. Researchers at St. Louis University have found that alkaline diets improved physical fitness of individuals in comparison to acidic diets. Improving your exercise performance can translate into greater weight loss and more energy.

Alkalinity Maintains Lean Muscle Mass and Youthfulness

Muscle tissue is the most metabolically active tissue in the body, so with more muscle, you burn more calories, even at rest. Unfortunately, as we age, we lose muscle mass. Loss of muscle decelerates your metabolism, and you're more likely to gain weight. You're also at a greater risk of falls and fractures; muscle loss can render you unsteady on your feet.

An alkaline diet protects muscle. A study that looked at a diet rich in potassium and magnesium (ample in fruits and vegetables), as well as a reduced acid load, found it preserved muscle in women. The researchers note: "Although protein is important for maintenance of muscle mass, eating fruits and vegetables that supply adequate amounts of potassium and magnesium are also relevant. The results suggest a potential role for diet in the prevention of muscle loss." Studies have also shown that a higher intake of foods rich in vitamin K (fruits and vegetables) is associated with more lean muscle. You will feel more energetic and more youthful, and you'll notice fine lines and wrinkles diminish.

Alkalinity Prevents Magnesium Deficiency

The fourth-most-abundant mineral in the body, magnesium is in charge of more than three hundred essential functions. It helps maintain normal nerve and muscle function, a normal heart rhythm, ideal blood pressure, and a healthy immune system. Magnesium is also involved in activating vitamin D, which is necessary for healthy bones, weight loss, immunity, heart health, blood sugar control, protection against cancer, and more.

Several studies have noted that women with osteoporosis have lower magnesium levels than those without. This is because magnesium regulates calcium absorption. Magnesium deficiencies also result in anxiety and sleep issues, headaches, and other negative side effects.

Many of us are deficient in this essential mineral, for two reasons: our foods are grown in magnesium-depleted soils, and high acid diets tend to siphon magnesium from the body. Fortunately, a diet high in alkaline foods supplies a healthy amount of magnesium for our bodies to function at peak levels.

Alkalinity Reduces Pain

I have really felt this benefit myself when I've gone alkaline, and I've heard about it from my patients as well. As their bodies become more alkaline, women report to me that they have had less joint pain, menstrual discomfort, and inflammation. Studies support the fact that chronic acidosis is associated with persistent pain and inflammation, especially back pain.

Add this to the fact that our fascia, the connective tissue in our body, also has hormone receptors in it. Along comes the hormonal decline associated with peri- and postmenopause. There are fewer hormones available to enter the cells of the fascia, so it weakens, causing greater aches and pain as we get older.

But none of this has to happen. Take Darla, one of my Magic Menopause clients, who at age fifty-five was really limited in her activities due to serious knee and foot pain. She was contemplating surgery when she joined my program. Going Keto-Green and improving her natural hormone balance completely eliminated these symptoms in just a few weeks.

Alkalinity Improves Detoxification

It can be a dirty environment out there—and inside our bodies too. Fortunately, our bodies are good housekeepers, automatically doing the job of cleaning out or neutralizing toxins through the colon, liver, kidneys, lungs, lymph system, and skin. Still, our bodies can get overloaded with undesirable things like mucus, old fecal matter, mineral deposits, toxic chemicals, bacteria, mycotoxins (mold-related substances), and more—all of which accumulate in various organs and tissues, affecting their operation. For this reason, we need to detoxify periodically.

An alkaline diet is effective for detoxification. Alkaline foods, such as fruits and vegetables, are great detoxifiers of the body, whereas acid foods are inflammatory and mucus-forming. Acids can morph into free radicals, causing tissue damage. When you eat more alkaline foods, they cool and soothe inflamed tissue, heal ulcerations, and enhance cellular functions. In short, they promote cleansing of toxins from the body.

This will keep you from getting the keto flu, which is partly a detox reaction.

How We're Going to Fix Your Hormones

At five feet eight inches tall, I maintain a weight of 150 pounds (as mentioned, I once weighed 240). I have four daughters and a busy family life, I run online programs for women and a foundation in honor of my son, and I lecture regularly around the country and world, training physicians. Yet I manage to stay healthy and at my ideal weight (or close to it, depending on my stress levels) by following the principles of the Hormone Fix.

It works at any stage of your life by merging all the benefits of a healthy keto diet with those of an alkaline diet, as well as incorporating important lifestyle strategies. To sum up, during menopause and other periods of hormonal change, this program can help balance your hormones, aid in weight loss, enhance your sex drive, increase your energy levels, help you sleep better, and reduce inflammation.

Balance Your Hormones

We'll dive more deeply into this in the next chapter, but suffice it to say that the unique combination of keto and alkaline foods optimizes three key hormones—insulin, cortisol, and oxytocin—so that you experience fewer symptoms like hot flashes and mood swings. If they do occur, they're usually shorter and less troublesome. As you balance these three hormones, your many other hormones come into balance more quickly.

Drop Pounds and Inches

As many of my patients and clients can attest, weight loss is a serious challenge during menopause. The Keto-Green Diet optimizes the hunger-regulating hormones leptin (satiety hormone) and ghrelin (hunger hormone), normalizes insulin and cortisol (two fat-storing hormones), and eliminates cravings so you can lose weight and comfortably keep it off.

Enhance Your Libido

The diet is rich in healthy fats, which improve the absorption of fat-soluble vitamins. This is especially true for vitamin D, a necessity for healthy function of your sex hormones. It also will improve your lipid profile, while helping balance testosterone and the other hormones depleted by menopause. Results: increased libido and more spark between the sheets!

Stop Energy Drain

Menopause can often leave you feeling fatigued and wiped out. My Keto-Green Diet helps maintain steady energy levels because healthy fats and ketones provide a clean, efficient energy source and support healthy hormone levels, especially when combined with an alkaline diet.

Reclaim Quality Sleep

When your diet is filled with sugar and carbohydrates (even those seemingly innocent 100-calorie fruit snack packs can spike and crash your blood sugar), your sleep is impacted. When you combine a high-carb diet with hot flashes, restless legs, heart palpitations, and other menopausal symptoms, your sleep can really suffer. The Keto-Green Diet balances blood sugar levels and optimizes hormones to improve sleep and reset your circadian rhythm—the body clock in which our physiological processes are synced to the twenty-four-hour solar cycle of light and dark.

Soothe Chronic Inflammation

When you cut your finger, the redness and swelling around the wound are signs of inflammation. This short-term type of inflammation, known as acute inflammation, is beneficial because it means your immune system is responding to injury and intruders, such as bacteria, in order to heal your body.

With chronic inflammation, your immune system fails to shut down. Instead, it releases a continuous stream of inflammatory substances that damage cells and accelerate aging. This deadly form of inflammation can increase during menopause, sparking unpleasant symptoms like chronic pain and playing a significant role in nearly every disease on earth. My Keto-Green Diet counters acidosis and inflammation and may reduce joint pain, back pain, and other inflammatory conditions, as many women in my programs and on this diet have experienced.

So get ready, feel encouraged, and claim your sexy youthfulness! You no longer need to accept hot flashes, low libido, brain fog, and other miseries of hormone imbalance. You hold tremendous power over your health and your quality of life. In all my years of researching and working with women (and men) on nutrition and hormone-reset programs, my Keto-Green approach is the best way I have found to get healthy, balance hormones, boost your energy and mood, become a highly efficient fat-burner, feel sexy again, and have loving relationships. What's not to love about that?

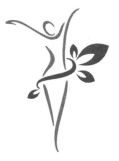

PART TWO

. . . .

The Keto-Green Diet

Chapter 4

Getting Started

Yes, it is time to get started. And remember, it doesn't have to be done perfectly; there is no failure here. It is about taking your next right step, one at a time, and just that positive action leads you to success. You now understand the role of your hormones in how badly you've been feeling and why you are experiencing peri- or postmenopausal symptoms. You also now see how the combination of ketogenic eating and alkalinizing your body greatly helps reduce those symptoms. In other words, you're ready to go!

It's now time to fix your hormones, ease those symptoms, lose weight, control your insatiable cravings, feel more energetic, improve your digestion, and more. To do that, you'll kick things off with the 10-Day Keto-Green Quick Start Detox. The feeling of empowerment that comes from fixing your hormones is just ten days away.

I've taken thousands of women through this ten-day process (followed by the twenty-one-day Keto-Green eating plan in Chapter 6) with wonderful outcomes. Their self-assessment questionnaires and lab results reveal the positive health changes behind their feelings: lower inflammation, improved adrenal gland functioning, normalized progesterone, better blood glucose control, and more. As a result, I often hear, "I haven't felt this good in decades!" Or "I don't even remember ever feeling this good!" And "I actually like myself again!"

I remember one woman, eighty-two-year-old Cheryl. She lived in a house beside a pond and had a rowboat in her backyard that she had not used in seven years. After doing the ten-day plan, Cheryl put that boat in the water and started rowing like crazy. Amazing! Her success and the successes of my other patients can be yours too—once you do the ten-day Quick Start.

Detoxifying Your Hormones

This Quick Start is a detox plan. I know that many people hear "detoxify" or "detoxification" and immediately think of a drug or alcohol detox, or even a regimen of water and juices. My plan is none of these. On the contrary, it involves delicious foods and smoothies—five days of an alkalinizing and cleansing diet, followed by five more days in which you induce fat-burning ketosis while continuing to stay alkaline. So over the next ten days, you'll give your body a break—a real rest and reset that will build the solid foundation for disease prevention for the rest of your life.

Detoxification is vital. On a daily basis, you are exposed to chemicals and toxins of all kinds, and it is high time to clean these out. Many of these toxins have been disrupting your natural hormone balance for decades. They enter your body through pesticides, herbicides, plastics, food, water, skin care products, direct exposure, and air. Once there, they mimic hormones such as estrogen, causing a disruption in your natural hormonal balance by affecting hormone communication and signaling.

This toxic assault taxes your liver and kidneys, both of which try desperately to break down these toxins and get them out of the body. But it's tough. Toxins do a lot of damage fairly quickly. For one thing, they significantly affect the trillions of healthy bacteria in the gut (the microbiome), which should be working to metabolize nutrients, make vitamins, and especially detoxify harmful forms of estrogen that you are exposed to from the metabolism of our own estrogens or from the environment. Toxic forms of estrogen can increase our risk of breast cancer, endometriosis, infertility, and autoimmune diseases. When you've been subjected to this stew of toxic chemicals and hormone disruptors, you often have severe problems with digestion, metabolism, and inflammation. Other manifestations of toxic exposure include worsening PMS symptoms, early symptoms of approaching menopause (such as hot flashes and mood swings), a tougher transition through menopause, and greater odds of hormone-related cancers. These toxins negatively affect our genetics and can cause DNA adducts—mutations in genes that result from exposure to specific carcinogens and lead to cancer.

The problems don't end there. An imbalance in your gut microbiota can increase levels of an enzyme called beta-glucuronidase, which in turn triggers reabsorption of estrogen back into circulation. This leads to estrogen dominance, a condition in which you have insufficient progesterone to balance the effects of estrogen in your body. Symptoms include breast swelling and tenderness, cramps, bloating, headaches or migraines, irritability, anxiety, depression, food cravings, brain fog, sleep difficulties, and lowered libido.

HEALTHY METABOLISM OF ESTROGEN

Estrogen is metabolized by your liver. It converts excess estrogen into breakdown products that can be eliminated from the body. Within the liver there are three main pathways through which estrogen can be metabolized. I compare these to the three rivers that encircle St. Simon's Island, Georgia (where I live), and flow into the Atlantic Ocean. Two of these rivers—the Satilla and the Altamaha Rivers—are quite polluted due to paper mills and other industries. The Georgia Department of Natural Resources samples fish from water bodies each year to test for contaminants such as PCBs, chlordane, and mercury, and has determined that you can't safely eat fish from the Satilla or Altamaha more than once a week (and for some types of fish, only once per month). The third, the Sapelo River, is not polluted and therefore great for recreation and fishing.

Like those first two rivers, there are two estrogen pathways that are toxic and unhealthy; and like the Sapelo River, the third pathway is healthier and preferred. That third pathway is called the 2-methyl-hydroxy pathway. If the body can convert estrogens along it, you will be healthier and reduce your risk of cancer. But if your body converts along the 16-alpha-hydroxy pathway or the 4-hydroxy pathway, you have a greater risk of cancer. These pathways can be assessed by urine or blood testing. (For more information, see the Resources.) Don't worry about remembering the chemical names of all the pathways. Just remember that the 2-methyl-hydroxy pathway is healthy and can be supported by detoxifying your body, eating probiotic rich foods, and including certain types of vegetables (methyl-group-containing veggies) in your diet.

Without getting too technical, methyl groups are made up of just a single carbon molecule with three hydrogen molecules surrounding it. Nutrients high in methyl groups include vitamin B12, folate, vitamin B6, choline, and the amino acids methionine and betaine. These nutrients support a process in which these methyl groups are added to proteins, DNA, homocysteine, and other molecules to keep your body detoxifying and functioning well. This is called methylation. Think of methylation like the spark plug in your car—it stimulates these reactions. Your body undertakes methylation billions of times in a single second. A breakdown in this process increases risks for infertility, osteoporosis, cancer, cervical dysplasia, depression, and dementia. Vegetables with methylation-supporting nutrients are the very same foods that are high in B vitamins, such as leafy green vegetables, fruits, whole grains, beans, peas, lentils, sunflower seeds, and nuts. Animal foods like egg yolk, chicken, turkey, fish, beef, pork, lamb, and liver also provide methyl groups.

Your Quick Start Guidelines

There's no way around this news: in order to begin fixing your hormones, you're going to need to eliminate a few things from your nutritional repertoire. But take heart, because you can return some of these foods and drinks to your lineup after the initial ten-day Quick Start. That said, many women report that they don't *want* these things once they've taken them out of their diet. You too may find that your taste for these things has diminished once you've detoxified and stabilized your hormones. Also, remember that what you eat is only part of it; the lifestyle hacks that I talk about at the end of the book are another part. Let's get started!

Do Away with Sugar

Sugar has a big impact on hormones. If you're eating sugar (whether natural sugars or artificial sweeteners), then your hormones are being affected on a daily basis. If you've been eating sugar all your life, then it possibly affected your ability to conceive, your ability to stay at an ideal weight, and even your ability to breeze through menopause. Sugar has a direct effect on hormonal conditions such as polycystic ovary syndrome. Too much sugar is also a strong inducer of inflammation, so it's a definite no-no for most of us, especially as we get older. Last, sugar also numbs the brain's sensor that prevents overeating. This means that your brain effectively stops releasing hormones like oxytocin to signal that you're full, and you're more likely to continue eating.

If you just can't imagine life without sugar in your coffee or tea, replace sugar with a bit of monkfruit-based sweetener, stevia, or xylitol. Cinnamon and pure vanilla extract can also satisfy a sweet tooth. Yes, my southern belles, say "no thank you" to sweet tea!

Let me add that fruit is a source of the sugar fructose, and too much fructose is not helpful for hormone balance. For this reason, you avoid fruit on my Quick Start plan.

Say No to Diet Sodas

You've heard that diet drinks aren't good for you, but how bad could they be? For one thing, diet sodas are high in phosphoric acid, which increases your risk of bone fracture. On the pH scale, most diet sodas come in at between 2.38 and 4.75—acidic enough to dissolve the enamel on your teeth! Your body has to neutralize the acid you just drank. It does so by extracting calcium from your bones. This leads to low bone-mineral density and the potential for breakage. In fact, women who drink three or more cola-based sodas daily have almost 4 percent less bone-mineral density in their hips than non-soda-drinkers.

Second, the artificial sweeteners in diet sodas cause weight gain. The physiological reasons behind this are not yet completely understood, but we know that there are sweet taste receptors in the mouth that send a "Calories are coming!" message to other parts of the body. The body starts turning on its digestive process, secreting more insulin, and stimulating hunger hormones—all of which signal the body to eat more and store more fat. Artificial sweeteners also trigger insulin resistance, making us put on fat. Bottom line: cut out the diet soda. (And cut out regular soda too!)

Get Off Gluten and Grains

Gluten is a protein found in wheat, rye, barley, malt, brewer's yeast, and sometimes oats. It also hides in the craziest places: chewing gum, some condiments (especially soy sauce), salad dressings, flavored coffees, snack foods, canned soups, a lot of processed foods, and some lunch meats (to keep them moist longer).

Gluten-containing foods can interfere with digestive health and eventually gut bacteria. They've been proven to trigger inflammation, heartburn, autoimmune disorders, neurological and behavioral issues, skin issues, osteoporosis, chronic fatigue, and other conditions.

It wasn't always this way. Gluten is not the same as it was decades ago. That's because modern farming practices have blended varieties of wheat to create hybrids that grow faster, yield more, are more resistant to insects, and create fluffier bread and grain foods. But they are also higher in gluten. The American way has been to eat cereal for breakfast, sandwiches for lunch, and rolls at dinner—and hence we are taking in a lot of gluten. Our digestive systems just can't handle that much of it. Gluten-containing foods are eliminated on the Quick Start. But don't worry. You'll enjoy your break from gluten and reap the benefits.

AGAINST THE GRAIN: MYCOTOXINS IN FOOD

Another reason to reduce or eliminate grains is because of mycotoxins. Some of the most prevalent toxins in the environment, mycotoxins are chemicals produced by fungi that often contaminate grains, nuts, beans, fruit, and coffee beans. Breathed in or ingested via food, mycotoxins cause symptoms such as weakened immunity, fever, pneumonia-like symptoms, heart disease, asthma, sinusitis, cancer, memory loss, vision loss, chronic fatigue, skin rashes, depression, ADHD, anxiety, and liver damage.

There are many different types of mycotoxins. One very interesting form, zearalenone (ZEN), is considered a "mycoestrogen." This means it has a molecular structure similar to estrogen. It can activate estrogen receptors and create reproductive system changes in both animals and humans.

ZEN has been used since 1969 in the U.S. cattle industry to boost animal growth rates, but it has been banned by the European Union. It has also been linked to breast enlargement in humans. In the body, ZEN has been shown to promote breast cancer cell growth in estrogen-receptor-positive cancers. It is also now connected to precocious puberty (puberty that begins before age eight) in girls.

ZEN is found in grain products including breakfast cereal, bread, pasta, beer, and processed foods—more reasons to leave wheat, barley, and corn out of your diet.

Ease Off Certain Beverages

I'm not going to recommend that you give up coffee. With a pH of 5, black coffee is less acidic than soda. It also contains high levels of antioxidants your body can easily absorb. But I am going to recommend that you keep your intake to one cup a day. Too much caffeine triggers an upswing in cortisol and other stress hormones, which has a weight gain effect, as I've explained. Green tea is a great substitute for coffee, so you might want to drink it exclusively, or just as a substitute for your usual second cup of coffee. It contains a little less caffeine, while providing lots of antioxidants. This may explain why the green-tea-drinking Japanese enjoy low levels of cancer despite their high incidence of smoking.

Another beverage to watch is alcohol. It's a depressant and generally high in sugar too. Plus alcohol relaxes your inhibitions, making it tough to stay on a healthy detoxifying diet through the whole ten days.

You may have heard that a glass of red wine a day is good for you because of the heart-healthy antioxidant resveratrol—and that's been proven. However, I believe that drinking wine while experiencing the fun and joy of being with friends and family produces more oxytocin, and that is the real elixir of longevity. You can get the same oxytocin burst, though, without the wine. So forgo your usual cabernet or chardonnay during the next ten days. Instead, check out my Kool Keto Mocktail, on page 302. For that occasional adult beverage, I do have some good news: tequila and potato vodka do not cause a significant increase in blood glucose and insulin—see my favorite indulgence, my Te-Keto Cocktail, on page 301. And know that you'll be able to ease it back in for days eleven to twenty-one.

Stay Hydrated

When you are well hydrated, you're less hungry (thirst can often be disguised as hunger). Staying hydrated allows your kidneys to get rid of toxins and helps your liver to more effectively metabolize fat.

As surgeons, we are taught that "the solution to pollution is dilution," and this is all the more important as you are detoxing. So how much is enough? One way to judge is by looking at the color of your urine. It should be clear (unclouded) and a very light yellow. A general rule of thumb: each day you should be drinking (between meals) approximately half your body weight in ounces of water. This is probably better based on your ideal weight, not your actual weight. For example, if your ideal weight is 140 pounds, you should drink 70 ounces of water daily, which amounts to about six 12-ounce bottles. Use common sense, though—if you're a marathoner running in the heat, you need more, and if you're a sedentary worker indoors, you probably need less.

But . . . Drink Less Water with Your Meals

When we ingest food, digestive juices pour into our stomachs. Drinking fluids dilutes these important juices, as well as the enzymes required for good digestion. If you want to drink with your meal, limit your intake to about 4 ounces. Ideally, you'll stop drinking twenty minutes prior to your meal and resume drinking two hours afterward. After a simple salad or smoothie, waiting 1 hour is typically long enough. The purest water choice is filtered water. Drink plenty of it between meals.

Chew Your Food Well

Chewing very thoroughly helps saliva break down your food. This eases digestion because food can then move through your system more easily, helping to prevent heartburn and embarrassing gas. It will also help you naturally limit your intake because you'll be better able to recognize your body's fullness signals.

I recommend that you chew each bite twenty to thirty times. When my daughter Amira was eight, she told me that chewing a grape so many times was really hard. Of course, she's right about that—obviously a single grape doesn't need that many chews! But give this practice a try. It can become a mindfulness practice that teaches you to fully enjoy your food. Not only that, you'll discover how well chewing allows your food to dissolve and digest.

Quick Start Detoxifying Foods

Here's a quick overview of what you'll eat for the next ten days:

Mostly alkaline foods. You'll be consuming a diet that is essentially 80 percent alkaline and 20 percent acidic (the suggested daily meal plans starting on page 92 show you how). Diets that are alkaline decrease inflammation, improve immune response, and assist with detoxification and fat loss.

Foods that detoxify harmful estrogens. Many of us need to eat more cruciferous vegetables such as broccoli, cauliflower, Brussels sprouts, and cabbage. These veggies contain influential plant chemicals, namely indole-3 carbinol (I3C) and diindolylmethane (DIM), that detoxify harmful estrogen molecules. Cruciferous veggies also release sulfur-containing nutrients that help the liver detoxify and block cancer cell formation.

Foods that are anti-inflammatory. Included in the Quick Start are foods high in omega-3 fats: organic grass-fed beef, organic poultry, and wild-caught salmon. Plant-based fats such as avocados, coconut oil, and olive oil are all potent anti-inflammatory foods, as well as hormone-balancing. So are nuts like almonds and Brazil nuts and seeds such as flaxseeds and chia seeds.

Foods that offer liver-detoxifying nutrients. Onions, garlic, and scallions are rich in sulfur-containing amino acids that not only are prebiotic foods but also help the liver detoxify more efficiently and reduce the production of excess estrogen. Delicious herbs such as oregano, thyme, rosemary, and sage are loaded with nutrients that promote liver detoxification too. A particularly powerful detoxifying herb is turmeric. In a review study published in *The Journal of Laboratory Automation* in 2016, researchers pointed out that curcumin, the active ingredient in turmeric, has a potent ability to destroy estrogen-receptor-positive cancer cells (most commonly found in breast cancer).

Foods that control insulin and blood sugar levels. Excess insulin in the bloodstream sets in motion a process in the body that overproduces estrogens, which can float around and enter target tissues. Limiting your intake of carbohydrates and getting into ketosis helps prevent this.

A daily Keto-Green smoothie. Each day, you'll enjoy a delicious, quick, easy-to-make smoothie that gets you alkaline in the morning because it's full of greens, healthy fats, and other alkalinizing ingredients. See recipes starting on page 208.

Bone broth. Another integral part of the Quick Start is bone broth (or, for vegetarians, an alkaline broth). It is so alkalinizing, full of hormone-balancing minerals, and supportive of balanced hormones and overall health. It helps with digestion, joint function, immunity, skin (it's loaded with collagen), and virtually every other function in the body. It's also high in magnesium, which most of us are deficient in. Everything from blood pressure to energy depends on magnesium, so giving your body more of it is a good idea. The best part is that bone broth is supereasy to make; see page 228 for the recipe. You can also purchase it.

Supplements. Because the body is designed to heal itself and be healthy—that's what it wants to do—I recommend helping it along with dietary supplements. See page 81 for a simple list and for advice on reading labels and choosing wisely.

The 10-Day Keto-Green Quick Start Detox Food List

What follows is a list of the many foods you can eat over the next ten days. This list is reprinted at the back of the book on a page you can more easily tear out and bring with you to the grocery store as a shopping list.

As much as possible, please choose organic, fresh whole foods and protein sources that are wild caught over farm raised, free range over caged, and grass fed over grain fed.

Alkaline Vegetables That Detoxify Estrogen

Bok choy
Broccoli
Brussels sprouts
Cabbage
Cauliflower

Greens: arugula, beet greens, kale, chard, collard, and mustard greens
Maca

Other Alkaline Vegetables

Alfalfa sprouts
Asparagus, green
Avocado (I know it's a fruit ☺)
Bamboo shoots
Bell peppers
Carrots
Celery
Cucumber
Eggplant
Greens: lettuces, spinach, and so forth
Jalapeño
Kimchi
Mushrooms
Onions
Scallions
Seaweed: all types, including nori
Snow peas
Tomatoes
Yellow squash
Zucchini

Protein Choices

Eggs, large, organic, and cage-free
Goat cheese
Organic chicken and turkey
Organic grass-fed beef
Pancetta or bacon (nitrate/nitrite free)
Protein powder, including collagen or vegetarian protein powder
    (such as pea and rice protein; choose one with less than 3 grams
    sugar per serving)

Shellfish: shrimp, scallops, or oysters
Tofu, miso, or tempeh (see vegan swaps on page 77)
White fish, such as rainbow trout, tilapia, or sea bass

Liver-Detoxifying Foods and Herbs

Artichoke hearts
Onions, garlic, and scallions
Oregano
Rosemary
Sage
Thyme

Other Quick Start Foods

Bone broth (see page 228 for recipe)
Vegetable or alkaline broth (see page 229 for recipe)

Oils and Vinegars

Apple cider vinegar (unfiltered)
Avocado oil
Coconut oil
MCT oil
Olive oil, extra-virgin
Organic ghee or butter (from grass-fed cows)
Rice or coconut vinegar
Sesame oil
Walnut oil

Herbs and Spices

Allspice
Basil, fresh or dried
Bay leaves
Black pepper, ground

Chives, fresh
Cilantro
Cinnamon sticks
Dry mustard
Garlic powder
Ginger root, fresh
Lemons
Limes
Mint, fresh or dried
Paprika
Parsley, fresh or dried
Red pepper flakes
Sea salt
Tarragon, fresh or dried

Nuts and Seeds

Almond or cashew butter
Almonds
Chia seeds
Flaxseeds
Pistachios
Pumpkin seeds
Sesame seeds
Sunflower seeds
Walnuts

Teas

Chai
Chamomile
Cinnamon
Green tea
Mushroom tea
Other herbal teas

Additional

Almond flour
Capers
Coconut aminos
Coffee
Full-fat whipping coconut cream
Kalamata olives
Maca, powdered, or Mighty Maca Plus
Nutritional yeast
Red curry sauce
Roasted red peppers, jarred
Tahini
Tamari sauce, preferably low-sodium

VEGAN SWAPS

Many people are eating less meat—whether to improve their health, the environment, or their budget. If you're among them, here are some substitutes you can make for animal foods and still stay Keto-Green. I recommend following the ten-day plan as closely as possible and use these swaps for the twenty-one-day plan.

Tofu, miso, or tempeh (non-GMO)

Vegetable burgers

Beans and lentils sparingly

Hummus

Nuts

Vegan protein powder (choose one with less than 3 grams sugar per serving)

Hemp hearts

Portobello mushrooms

The Day 6 Upgrade: Keto-Green Fasting

After five days of Quick Start detoxing, you'll be ready to ramp up to a form of intermittent fasting, in which you will go fifteen hours between dinner and breakfast without food. Since this is overnight, much of this fast happens when you wouldn't be eating anyway—when you're sleeping. Simply have your dinner before 7 P.M., preferably by 5 P.M. After, you can enjoy one cup of tea if you'd like in the evening. This limited fluid will ensure your digestive enzymes stay concentrated and you will be less likely to get up in the middle of the night to use the bathroom. Then during the day, the window in which you eat is roughly a nine-hour period.

On day 8, however, I recommend a one-day liquid fast to empower your detoxification and increase ketosis. You'll have green smoothies, water, and bone broth, so you really won't go hungry! You can also make this day a water fasting day, with your physician's approval.

Keto-Green fasting pushes you into ketosis faster, forces the body to get energy by converting tough-to-budge fat into ketones and find energy reserves beyond stored glucose (thus burning fat), and prevents the need for frequent urination during the night. Besides helping you shed pounds, ketones keep your blood sugar and insulin levels steady, which is why you'll often feel more energetic with this type of fasting.

Your body will welcome the opportunity to fast. Evolution-wise, our bodies were programmed long ago to withstand periods of fasting. This pattern of eating dates back to ancient times, when people depended on the natural cycles of daylight and nighttime, with food primarily eaten during the day and fasting occurring at night.

A growing body of research suggests that intermittent fasting and time-restricted feeding bestow other powerful health benefits. Take a look.

Fasting Prevents Breast Cancer

In one study, breast cancer survivors who typically didn't eat for at least twelve and a half hours overnight had a 36 percent reduction in the risk of their breast cancer returning, compared with those who had shorter overnight fasts.

Fasting Cleans Defective Cells

Intermittent fasting kick-starts autophagy. This is a process by which the body gets rid of cells that have a greater risk of becoming infected or cancerous. These are cells that also lead to accelerated aging, Alzheimer's disease, and type 2 diabetes. Think of autophagy like spring cleaning—it tosses out the junk and clears the way for health and vitality.

Eating, however, prevents autophagy. Even a little food triggers an enzyme called mTOR, a powerful inhibitor of autophagy. Too much mTOR can lead to obesity, diabetes, and neurodegenerative diseases. Low levels of mTOR have been found to decrease cancer risk, decrease inflammation, and improve insulin sensitivity, and may also increase longevity. This is why intermittent and prolonged fasting is important for good health.

Fasting Creates a Healthy Gut and Circadian Rhythm

Inside the gut are trillions of healthy bacteria (the microbiome). They are affected not only by what we eat but also by when we eat. In a study published in the scientific journal *Cell*, researchers discovered that gut bacteria have their own circadian rhythm, like humans have—a clock of sorts, in which our physiological processes are synced to the twenty-four-hour solar cycle of light and dark. For example, your body starts to wind down and prepare for sleep after sunset, and it's programmed to wake up at sunrise.

When the microbiome's circadian rhythm is thrown off, there's trouble: brain fog, slower metabolism, insulin resistance, inability to burn fat, and impaired detoxification. What disrupts the microbiome's rhythm? Erratic eating patterns, eating all day, and night eating. Fortunately, time-restricted feeding, such as Keto-Green fasting, restores normal gut circadian rhythms and prevents these complications. In other words, intermittent fasting lets your digestive tract "rest and digest." Giving your digestion a break can also help to heal any damage that you may have done to your gut lining over the years. Remember too that a healthy gut promotes healthy estrogen metabolism.

Fasting Resolves Insulin Resistance

Other studies have found that intermittent fasting helps prevent insulin resistance (which, as you know by now, triggers hot flashes and other menopause symptoms) and enhances hormone function that helps with weight loss, including the loss of belly fat. Keto-Green fasting is thus an excellent way to turn up hormone-balancing a few more notches!

Fasting Keeps Fat Off for Good

Many of us are used to cutting calories to lose weight. But the problem with calorie restriction is that it forces the metabolism to slow down to the lowered calorie intake. If you return to eating a higher amount of calories after the diet, your now slower metabolism makes weight regain inevitable.

Unlike calorie restriction, fasting does not cause weight regain, because during fasting you switch fuel sources from food to stored fat.

Studies have directly compared daily caloric restriction to intermittent fasting. In a 2016 study published in the journal *Obesity,* researchers compared zero-calorie alternate-day fasting (a form of intermittent fasting) with daily caloric restriction in obese adults.

What were the findings? Fat loss in the trunk, which includes the more dangerous fat packed in around the organs, was almost twice as high with fasting as opposed to calorie cutting. As for body fat, there was almost six times the amount of fat loss using fasting.

The study also addressed a big concern: does fasting burn up muscle? Well, the calorie restrictors lost a significant amount of muscle, but the fasters did not. As it turned out, fasting is *four times better* at preserving lean mass.

What about the effect of these protocols on metabolism? After all, that's what determines whether you can keep weight off. With calorie restriction, metabolism fell by 76 calories a day. Using fasting, it dropped only 29 calories a day. Do the math: *Daily caloric reduction causes almost two and a half times as much metabolic slowdown as fasting!*

FASTING: ITS BENEFITS FOR WOMEN

In addition to the benefits of fasting I've described, there are other pluses—and best of all, they apply specifically to women. These compelling benefits were enumerated in a scientific review published in 2016 in *The Journal of Mid-Life Health*. Fasting can:

- Reduce body weight
- Slow down the growth of tumors and decrease cancer risk
- Manage symptoms of polycystic ovary syndrome (PCOS)
- Improve joint and bone health
- Help manage blood sugar
- Protect the heart (particularly intermittent fasting)
- Reduce risk for menstrual problems
- Improve mental health during menopause transition
- Reduce symptoms of anxiety and depression
- Ease stress levels

I also feel that the upsurge in autoimmune diseases is the result of the constant layering of toxins and demands on our bodies without sufficient time for the body to rest. Fasting allows resting and repair, and quite possibly helps prevent or even reverse these illnesses—for free!

Supplementing Your Diet

I am frequently asked for my opinion on supplements. My position is simple and unequivocal: I recommend them! I've spent a lot of time studying and researching the quality, bioavailability, sustainability, and efficacy of various supplements and am therefore very particular about what I recommend. (For what I consider the "gold standard" for supplements, see the Resources section.)

Generally, you can support your energy, detoxification, fat-burning, and hormone balance with the following supplements:

A multivitamin/mineral. This lays an important foundation. By filling gaps in today's nutrient-depleted food, a multivitamin provides nutritional insurance. Many people also have nutrient deficiencies that put them at a hormonal disadvantage. If your body is lacking in zinc, iron, and B vitamins, for example, you may present symptoms of a hormonal imbalance such as polycystic ovary syndrome, infertility, or miscarriage. The body depends on an intricate balance of nutrients in order to get the reproductive processes working well.

There are many types of multis, and they are not all the same. The ones I recommend have a multivitamin/mineral blend featuring activated vitamins, including folate as 5-MTHF (5-methyltetrahydrofolate), and Albion chelated mineral complexes because these are well absorbed.

Recommended dosage: 2 tablets daily, 1 taken in the morning and 1 in the evening (preferably with food).

Omega-3 fish oil. The important components of fish oil are the omega-3 fatty acids EPA and DHA. In a 2009 study conducted in Canada, 120 women going through menopause were given either a fish oil supplement providing 1,200 milligrams of EPA and DHA or a placebo for two months. Prior to the study, these women averaged about 2.8 hot flashes daily. But after eight weeks, their hot flashes decreased by 55 percent in the EPA and DHA group, but by only 25 percent in the placebo group.

It's important to choose a high-quality fish oil that is certified by the International Fish Oils Standards (IFOS), guaranteeing quality, potency, and purity. Always look at the supplement facts information, which is broken down by the amount of EPA and DHA oils. A good omega-3 will have 360 milligrams EPA and 240 milligrams DHA per 1,000-milligram capsule. There are newer enzymatically treated omega-3 supplements that boast higher absorption; these are good, especially if you have digestive issues. And if you are worried about a fishy smell when you burp, look for enteric-coated capsules.

Recommended dosage: 1,000 milligrams (with 360 milligrams EPA and 240 milligrams DHA) taken once in the morning and in the evening.

Vitamin C. The human body does not make vitamin C, so it must be obtained through diet or supplements. Vitamin C supplementation boosts immunity, supports the adrenal glands, and enhances collagen formation for healthy skin. Vitamin C is also an important antioxidant that protects cells from heart disease and cancer.

Recommended dosage: Start with a daily dose of 500 to 2,000 milligrams, taken any time of the day. I typically recommend higher doses—4,000 milligrams a day—to women who have experienced frequent urinary tract infections.

Magnesium. This important mineral is essential for over three hundred cellular processes within our body, but too many of us are deficient in it. Indeed, in my own medical practice, 99 percent of patients over age forty have had suboptimal magnesium levels. Deficiencies—which are clearly all too common—can result in cramps, restless legs, palpitations, anxiety, constipation, sore muscles, sleep difficulties, moodiness, and other unpleasant symptoms.

Magnesium comes in many forms. While the most common type, magnesium citrate, is helpful in preventing constipation, our bodies don't absorb it all that well. Instead, I recommend magnesium malate—a combination of magnesium and malic acid, which supports energy production and may also support antioxidant systems by enhancing glutathione and antioxidant enzymes. Another good option is magnesium lysinate glycinate chelate, which is a highly soluble and easily absorbed form. To support brain health and cognitive function—if this is a priority for you—take the magnesium L-threonate form. It is the only form shown to cross the blood-brain barrier. I personally take this one regularly.

Recommended dosage: 250 milligrams (or up to 1,000 milligrams) taken before bedtime. (Back off the dose if you get loose stools.)

A probiotic. Probiotics are friendly bacteria in supplement form that empower a healthy gastrointestinal tract. Healthwise, probiotics benefit you by curbing the growth of harmful gut bacteria, promoting good digestion, boosting immune function, and increasing your resistance to infection.

Probiotics are equally powerful for healthy hormonal detoxification and even our moods. Sadly, though, these beneficial bugs are under constant assault from our environment, making it crucial to supplement with them as well as eat fermented foods (which are high in probiotics).

Recommended dosage: Typically, one dose of 30 billion CFUs (colony-forming units) taken before bedtime. If you have been diagnosed with small intestine bacterial overgrowth (SIBO), you must correct this condition prior to supplementing with probiotics.

PROBIOTIC PICKS

Probiotics (the word literally means "for life") consist of different strains of beneficial bacteria. Different strains produce different results, and many strains exist—which is why choosing a probiotic supplement can be confusing. Furthermore, when one probiotic strain has a certain health benefit, you can't assume that another strain has similar properties.

What I recommend is that you select a probiotic formulated with four of the most highly researched species: *Bifidobacterium lactis, Bifidobacterium longum, Lactobacillus acidophilus,* and *Lactobacillus plantarum.* Here is a summary of their specific benefits, based on extensive scientific research.

Bifidobacterium lactis

- Survives well in the acid environment of the stomach and gut
- Boosts immunity, thereby increasing resistance to illness and infection
- Is effective against constipation
- Helps reduce blood sugar

Bifidobacterium longum

- Survives well in the acid environment of the stomach and gut
- Helps reduce depression in people who suffer from irritable bowel syndrome (IBS)

- Binds with carcinogens to usher them from the body and help prevent colon cancer
- Reduces DNA damage that can trigger the development of malignant cells
- Can be used vaginally as well

Lactobacillus acidophilus

- Survives well in the acid environment of the stomach and gut
- Boosts immunity
- Colonizes well in the intestine, but also in the urethra, colon, and vagina (where it inhibits vaginal infections and boosts vaginal and bladder health)
- Reduces cholesterol
- Controls urinary tract infections
- Eases acne
- Reduces DNA damage that can trigger the development of malignant cells

Lactobacillus plantarum

- Survives well in the intestines
- Fights common germs
- Boosts the immune system

All four of these strains have a long history of safe use. Read labels to make sure that these strains are present and that the product contains live and active bacterial cultures. Also, take a supplement that contains 30 billion CFUs of these strains daily.

A liver detox supplement. If your Medical Symptom Toxicity Questionnaire score (see page 21) is above 20, I suggest you get yourself a liver support supplement containing the herb milk thistle. The active ingredient in milk thistle, silymarin, has therapeutic value in treating liver disorders, inflammatory conditions, cancer, neurological problems, skin diseases, and high cholesterol.

Recommended dosage: Follow the manufacturer's instructions and take in the morning, or before meals for an appetite-suppressant effect.

Fiber supplementation. For detoxification, to aid elimination, and as a prebiotic, it is important to add fiber-rich seeds, such as freshly ground flaxseeds, hemp seeds, and chia seeds, to your foods. Alternatively, you can take a fiber supplement. See the Resources section for recommendations.

Maca. Maca is an adaptogen, which means it can help support your adrenals, especially against the impact of burnout and chronic stress. Additionally, maca helps keep the body from being too acidic (stress is extremely acidifying by itself) because it is very alkalinizing. Maca also supports hormone balance, sex drive, and mood, and it decreases hot flashes.

Unfortunately, maca by itself doesn't taste so good! My preference is maca combined with other superfoods, as in my Mighty Maca Plus formula, mixed in water or added to a smoothie. Mighty Maca Plus contains superfoods from around the world, such as turmeric, resveratrol, quercetin, cat's claw herb, cinnamon, apple fiber, spirulina, and others. These have a potent combined antioxidant effect. Plus it tastes great! I have nearly ten years of clinical results and client testimonials praising the benefits clients have gotten with this combination of ingredients, from improvements in blood sugar control to a reduction in hot flashes, reduced cravings, improvement in aches and pains, better mood, increased libido, and more.

Recommended dosage: Follow the manufacturer's instructions and take in the morning as part of your Keto-Green Shake.

THE POWER OF MACA

I first learned about maca when I visited Peru. It's a radish-like tuber that grows above eleven thousand feet in the country's central highlands. Maca has long been an important staple for native Peruvians. Highly nutritious, the plant is rich in vitamins, minerals, protein, carbohydrates, fiber, amino acids, and fatty acids.

I experienced the healing power of maca myself. Each day, I drank it mixed in juice (because it tasted terrible in just water) while trying desperately to regain my footing, my fertility, and my life after my son died. I felt its benefits almost immediately—more energy, a better mood, and just feeling more like my old self.

It's one thing to experience benefits personally, but as a doctor and scientist, I researched with due diligence and found scientific research to prove that maca:

- Improves female reproductive hormone function
- Boosts memory
- Eases depression, anxiety, PMS, and other menopausal symptoms
- Improves libido
- Enhances energy and fights fatigue
- Helps in the treatment of osteoporosis and metabolic syndrome
- Reduces blood glucose levels
- Works as an antioxidant
- Lowers blood pressure
- Protects the liver and immune system
- Fights tumors
- Optimizes ovarian function

Chapter 5

The 10-Day Keto-Green Quick Start Detox

So here it is: your 10-Day Keto-Green Quick Start. As you can see, it includes three meals per day, with instructions for getting alkaline the first five days and into ketosis the next five. I've provided recipes in the back of the book, but there is flexibility to create your own meals from the food lists below, based on the foods you like. If you don't see a portion size given, feel free to eat as much as you like, but eat until you just feel satisfied, without feeling stuffed.

As you follow the Quick Start, you'll find yourself feeling more energetic, sleeping better, experiencing fewer symptoms, and losing weight (up to a pound a day)—all while enjoying delicious and nutritious foods.

Remember that this Quick Start is a tool that you can use periodically throughout the year for improved hormonal health and longevity. You can use it once a month, or at the start of each new season. Go back to the Quick Start if your weight starts creeping up, or if you need to slim down quickly for a special occasion.

CREATE YOUR QUICK START PLATE

80 percent alkalinizing vegetables and 20 percent protein

For the first five days, while you're focused on getting alkaline, an easy way to plan your lunches and dinners is to use your dinner plate as a guideline. Simply fill a little more than three-fourths of your plate (80 percent) with alkalinizing vegetables. In the remaining space, place your healthy protein and fat choices.

From day 6 to day 10, you'll simply add more healthy fats to create more of a keto-alkalinizing plate. For example, two-thirds of your plate might hold alkalinizing veggies, a middle circle holds healthy fats such as avocado, olives, or nuts and seeds, and the rest is filled with protein.

That's really all there is to it. The meal plans below will guide you, and pretty soon meal planning will be a cinch.

The First Five Days: Do This Every Day upon Awakening

- Test your urinary pH first thing in the morning (and periodically throughout the day), with the goal of keeping at or above 7.0. Record everything in your Daily Tracker. (See the Self-Tests section.)
- Drink a large glass of warm water to which you've added ½ teaspoon lemon juice, ½ to 1 tablespoon unfiltered apple cider vinegar, and 1 pinch cayenne pepper (to stimulate detox). If you are not alkaline, meaning that your urine pH is below 7.0 persis-

tently, add ½ teaspoon baking soda to the mix or mix the baking soda with water and drink to boost alkalinization.

- Enjoy a cup of coffee or tea (such as cinnamon, chamomile, chai, or green, with a cinnamon stick). I find that many women have undiagnosed dairy sensitivities, but even if that doesn't sound like your issue, it's a good idea to just go dairy free these first ten days. If you typically use a little splash of low-fat milk in your coffee, try unsweetened coconut or almond milk instead. Add 1 teaspoon ghee and/or 1 tablespoon MCT oil to boost your fat intake necessary for ketosis, also adding creaminess; blend it all together. This beverage will also stave off hunger and cravings.
- Begin your day with quiet time to meditate, pray, or express gratitude. Use your Daily Tracker to record your thoughts and feelings and set your intentions for the day.

MCT: A FAT-BURNING OIL

I'm partial to MCT oil, otherwise known as medium-chain triglyceride oil. It is a special type of fat derived from coconut or palm kernel oils that the body readily uses for energy. MCTs are the easiest fat for the body to convert into ketones, and they're less likely to be turned into body fat. In addition, MCT oil increases metabolism and appears to normalize low thyroid function, making it easier for the body to burn stored fat.

MCT oil is made from coconut oil, but don't confuse them as the same thing. There are four kinds of MCTs found in coconut oil: C6, C8, C10, and C12. (The numbers refer to the length of the carbon chains.) Among these, the most superior is C8, caprylic acid—and you should look for an oil that consists mostly of C8. It has the best ketone-producing and fat-burning profile. In fact, C8 is the fastest MCT to metabolize, and it bypasses liver processing entirely and is therefore less likely to be stored as body fat. Another benefit of C8 is that it helps support a healthy gut due to its powerful antimicrobial properties—it's able to eliminate harmful bacteria without interfering with good bacteria. It will improve the intestinal ecosystem and decreases leaky gut.

MCT oil can be used as a salad dressing and drizzled over vegetables.

DAY 1

BREAKFAST

Warm lemon water

Keto-Green Smoothie

Take your morning supplements

MIDMORNING

Drink regular small amounts of filtered water, totaling 32 ounces
(4 cups) prior to lunch

Sip 1 to 2 cups of tea (such as cinnamon, chamomile, chai, or green
with a cinnamon stick)

LUNCH*

Organic chicken or wild-caught fish

Fresh salad of greens and veggies, topped with sprouts and nuts,
drizzled with 1 to 2 tablespoons healthy oil such as olive oil,
walnut oil, or avocado oil, along with a few tablespoons of
vinegar (see salad dressing options in Recipes)

MIDAFTERNOON

Drink 32 ounces (4 cups) of filtered water

DINNER

Crock-Pot Chicken Soup

Cauliflower Mash

Take your evening supplements

---

* This lunch can be substituted for any lunch during the ten days.

DAY 2

BREAKFAST

Warm lemon water

Keto-Green Smoothie

Take your morning supplements

MIDMORNING

Drink regular small amounts of filtered water, totaling 32 ounces
(4 cups) prior to lunch

Sip 1 to 2 cups of tea (such as cinnamon, chamomile, chai, or green
with a cinnamon stick)

LUNCH

Almond or cashew butter with celery sticks and sliced cucumber, or
leftover *Crock-Pot Chicken Soup*

MIDAFTERNOON

Drink 32 ounces (4 cups) of filtered water

DINNER

Pistachio White Fish, or other white fish topped with tahini and
chopped pistachios

Steamed asparagus and side salad

Take your evening supplements

DAY 3

BREAKFAST

Warm lemon water

Keto-Green Smoothie

Take your morning supplements

MIDMORNING

Drink regular small amounts of filtered water, totaling 32 ounces
(4 cups) prior to lunch

Sip 1 to 2 cups of tea (such as cinnamon, chamomile, chai, or green
with a cinnamon stick)

LUNCH

Broccoli Slaw and Egg Salad, topped with ¼ cup chopped almonds

MIDAFTERNOON

Drink 32 ounces (4 cups) of filtered water

DINNER

Cruciferous Veggie Bake, topped with sliced avocado

Take your evening supplements

DAY 4

BREAKFAST

Warm lemon water

Keto-Green Smoothie

Take your morning supplements

MIDMORNING

Drink regular small amounts of filtered water, totaling 32 ounces
(4 cups) prior to lunch

Sip 1 to 2 cups of tea (such as cinnamon, chamomile, chai, or green
with a cinnamon stick)

LUNCH

Leftover *Cruciferous Veggie Bake* or *DIY Keto-Green Salad*

MIDAFTERNOON

Drink 32 ounces (4 cups) of filtered water

DINNER

Crock-Pot Roast Beef

Sautéed Beet Greens

Take your evening supplements

DAY 5

BREAKFAST
Warm lemon water
Keto-Green Shake
Take your morning supplements

MIDMORNING
Drink regular small amounts of filtered water, totaling 32 ounces
(4 cups) prior to lunch
Sip 1 to 2 cups of tea (such as cinnamon, chamomile, chai, or green
with a cinnamon stick)

LUNCH
Tuna Salad and Mayonnaise Stuffed Avocado

MIDAFTERNOON
Drink 32 ounces (4 cups) of filtered water

DINNER
Turkey Meatballs or *Nut and Seed No-Meat Balls with Zucchini
Noodles*
Easy Tomato Soup
Small green salad drizzled with 1 to 2 tablespoons healthy oil and a
few tablespoons of vinegar
Take your evening supplements

HACKS FOR GETTING AND STAYING ALKALINE

- Test, don't guess! Rather than assuming that you are
  alkaline, it is supereasy to check your urine pH so you
  know for sure. I recommend testing in the morning
  on rising, and then frequently throughout the day if
  you want. (On day 6, you'll start checking your
  ketones too.)

- Every morning, remember to drink a large glass of warm water to which you've added ½ teaspoon lemon juice, ½ to 1 tablespoon unfiltered apple cider vinegar, and 1 pinch cayenne pepper. Add ½ teaspoon baking soda if you are persistently acidic.
- Briefly cook or sauté your greens to help your body fully absorb their nutrients.
- Double the green veggies in your salad, and add sprouts to your Keto-Green Shake.
- Slow down your eating and chew your food even better.
- Drink extra bone broth (or alkaline broth—an option for vegans and vegetarians—that is made with alkalinizing vegetables only).
- Make sure you're hydrating your body properly with enough filtered water in between meals.
- Drink 1 teaspoon to 1 tablespoon apple cider vinegar before your meals to help digestion and alkalinity.
- Use MCT oil or EVOO (extra virgin olive oil) as the oil base in your salad dressings.
- Add a chelated mineral supplement to your supplement regimen. Take magnesium at bedtime.
- Constipation contributes to acidity—add a probiotic, magnesium, vitamin C, and a fiber supplement until you are having daily bowel movements. You can also increase MCT oil or add cod liver oil at a dosage of 1 tablespoon twice daily.
- Always buy quality. Especially when it comes to fat, buying free-range, grass-fed, non–genetically modified (GMO) foods becomes crucial. Whenever possible, choose organic, since conventional foods often grow in mineral-depleted, toxin-loaded soil.
- Don't try to be perfect. A confession I frequently hear is: "I had some red wine last night and, okay, some chocolate cake." I say, "Me too!" Not to worry: just get

right back on track. Real life happens, and to stay the course completely is rare. Last year I traveled to Poland, and I must admit that although I was able to stay Keto-Green most of the time due to the delicious whole foods available everywhere, I did quite a bit of feasting too. And yes, I confess that I had a chocolate pastry one morning for breakfast. Do your best, but give yourself a little leeway. The principles work! Keep at it.

- Look beyond diet. My program isn't just about food. Quality sleep becomes crucial to staying alkaline. Stress management, exercise, and healthy bowel movements all contribute. Oxytocin, that wonderful hormone released when you hug, love someone, or have an orgasm, also creates alkalizing benefits, so healthy relationships will help you stay alkaline too. The Keto-Green lifestyle will become a way of life you love, while tempering cortisol and improving insulin sensitivity—both keys to healthy longevity.

Days 6–10: Move into Ketosis

Do This Every Day upon Awakening

- Test your urinary pH first thing in the morning (and periodically throughout the day if you want), with the goal of keeping at or above 7.0. Note how it fluctuates and when. This is part of the discovery process. In addition to checking your urinary pH, check your urinary ketones with urine test strips (see Resources for my combined urine pH and ketone strips), or check blood ketones with a ketone monitor; the goal is to see positive ketones. (Again, testing is not mandatory but is very insightful.) Record everything in your Daily Tracker.

- Drink a large glass of warm water to which you've added ½ teaspoon lemon juice, ½ to 1 tablespoon unfiltered apple cider vinegar, and 1 pinch cayenne pepper. Add ½ teaspoon baking soda if you are not getting alkaline, meaning your urine pH is below 7.0.
- Sit quietly, meditate, pray, or express gratitude. Use your Daily Tracker to record your thoughts and feelings and to set your intentions for the day.
- Start Keto-Green fasting: Eat no later than 7 P.M. and drink no fluids overnight either, with the exception of having a glass of water or herbal tea after dinner. Work to keep thirteen to fifteen hours between dinner and breakfast. So if you finish dinner by 6:30 P.M., have your Keto-Green Smoothie between 7:30 and 9:30 A.M.
- As part of your morning routine, prepare *Keto Coffee* or *Tea* in order to further induce ketosis and manage cravings.
- Prepare a bone broth in advance and enjoy with any of the meals, if desired.

DAY 6

BREAKFAST

Warm lemon water

Keto-Green Smoothie

Take your morning supplements

MIDMORNING

Drink regular small amounts of filtered water, totaling 32 ounces
(4 cups) prior to lunch

Sip 1 to 2 cups of tea (such as cinnamon, chamomile, chai, or green
with a cinnamon stick)

LUNCH

Easy Keto Frittata with Sautéed Spinach

MIDAFTERNOON

Drink 32 ounces (4 cups) of filtered water

DINNER

Sautéed shrimp or scallops with stir-fry vegetables, or raw or
steamed oysters

Sautéed Beet Greens sprinkled with sesame seeds

Take your evening supplements

DAY 7

BREAKFAST

Warm lemon water

Keto-Green Shake

Take your morning supplements

MIDMORNING

Drink regular small amounts of filtered water, totaling 32 ounces
(4 cups) prior to lunch

Sip 1 to 2 cups of tea (such as cinnamon, chamomile, chai, or green
with a cinnamon stick)

LUNCH

Burger patty topped with kimchi (or sauerkraut) and sriracha
mayonnaise

MIDAFTERNOON

Drink 32 ounces (4 cups) of filtered water

DINNER

Oven-Roasted Ratatouille

Sliced avocado

Take your evening supplements

DAY 8

Today is a modified fasting day to empower your detoxification and increase ketosis. You can also make this day a water fasting day, with your physician's approval. You may still begin the day with a *Keto Coffee* or *Tea,* using 2 tablespoons of MCT oil, which will help stave off hunger. Remember, this increases autophagy and all the rejuvenating aspects that go with it.

BREAKFAST
Warm lemon water
Keto-Green Smoothie
Take your morning supplements

MIDMORNING
Drink regular small amounts of filtered water, totaling 32 ounces
  (4 cups) prior to lunch
Sip 1 to 2 cups of tea (such as cinnamon, chamomile, chai, or green
  with a cinnamon stick)

LUNCH
Bone Broth
Keto-Green Smoothie

MIDAFTERNOON
Drink 32 ounces (4 cups) of filtered water

DINNER
Bone Broth
Keto-Green Shake
Take your evening supplements

DAY 9

BREAKFAST

Warm lemon water

Continue the fast with *Keto Coffee* or *Tea* only

Take your morning supplements

MIDMORNING

Drink regular small amounts of filtered water, totaling 32 ounces (4 cups) prior to lunch

Sip 1 to 2 cups of tea (such as cinnamon, chamomile, chai, or green with a cinnamon stick)

You did it! You accomplished an approximately forty-hour modified extended fast. This helps speed the resetting of hormones. Next time you may want to try it with water only.

LUNCH

Smoked salmon topped with capers, onions, and sprouts, wrapped in nori or lettuce

Serve with a side salad or sautéed greens

MIDAFTERNOON

Drink 32 ounces (4 cups) of filtered water

DINNER

Bone Broth

Keto-Green Shake or *Easy Keto-Green Veggie Sauté* (page 262)

Take your evening supplements

This light dinner again is to further put you in a keto-alkaline state and increase insulin sensitivity and digestive system repair.

DAY 10

BREAKFAST

Warm lemon water

Keto-Green Shake or other Keto-Green breakfast option (see page 217)

Take your morning supplements

MIDMORNING

Drink regular small amounts of filtered water, totaling 32 ounces (4 cups) prior to lunch

Sip 1 to 2 cups of tea (such as cinnamon, chamomile, chai, or green with a cinnamon stick)

LUNCH

DIY Keto-Green Salad served with hard-boiled eggs, topped with broccoli sprouts and sunflower or pumpkin seeds; drizzle salad with 1 to 2 tablespoons MCT oil or EVOO, along with a few tablespoons of vinegar

MIDAFTERNOON

Drink 32 ounces (4 cups) of filtered water

DINNER

Spicy Chicken Stir-Fry (or substitute tempeh, beef, or fish for the chicken)

Take your evening supplements

THE NO-SNACK RULE

Do not eat between meals and do not snack. That advice might seem to fly in the face of conventional wisdom, but here's the truth: if you're over forty, snacking can be destructive to your goals. It can cause insulin resistance, weight gain, hot flashes, and inflammation. If you feel hunger pangs during the day, add more healthy fats, oils, and nuts to your meals. You can also increase your portion size. The hunger pangs will disappear. Eventually you'll retrain your body to not desire snacks at all.

Staying the Course

You might be thinking, "What happens if I get to day 6 and I go off the plan?" Great question—one that I hear all the time. My answer is to continue on and do the best you can, starting at the very next meal. I would love you to get an A-plus on this, but it's just as good to get a passing grade.

If you have been testing your urine but haven't gotten into ketosis or consistently alkaline, this plan is still working so stay with it. Often it may be because of a significantly stalled metabolism, candida or yeast, or high blood sugar and will take more time for some of us than others.

Above all, don't beat yourself up. Be kind to you. We women can be our own worst critics and talk down to ourselves and bash our bodies. I say, "Get that nasty witch off your shoulder!" Step outside yourself and think of yourself as another person—your daughter, your best friend, your mom. Would you say those things to them? Of course not! Dispense with self-talk that is judgmental and discouraging. Instead, talk to yourself with encouragement—be your own best friend and coach.

Chapter 6

Keto-Green for 21 Days

You are almost through or have just finished the 10-Day Keto-Green Quick Start Detox, and my hunch is that you feel lighter, look slimmer, and have more energy. That's because when you eat mainly Keto-Green foods and give your body a break from refined sugar, gluten, and processed carbs, your body sheds weight rapidly and your energy soars. The Quick Start improves insulin sensitivity, which means it's easier to turn the nutrients you eat into energy; it balances cortisol, so you feel less stressed; and it helps your body produce more feel-good oxytocin.

Also, because this plan detoxifies your system, your body's immune and digestive systems will be stronger and you will have a lower risk of getting ill. Finally, this detoxification regimen has begun to balance your hormones, so you feel more like yourself. Amazing, right? I hope you love your progress.

The 10-Day Keto-Green Quick Start Detox also paved the way to improved eating habits that will continue to fix your hormones, metabolism, and overall health. I know it's tempting to return to your old way of eating, but you don't want to miss out on the chance to lose more weight and feel even better. This is where my Keto-Green Diet comes in—a full twenty-one days of meal plans and recipes that expand your options and add protein to every meal. No more liquid-only meals now (though you can always do the Quick Start again when you feel you need it). This is a more lenient, everyday eating style.

Keto-Green Eating Made Easy

On the twenty-one-day plan, focus on the following:

- Get acquainted with alkaline and acid food choices (refer to the expanded lists starting on page 308). Keep your fridge stocked with the low-carbohydrate alkaline vegetables you enjoyed while detoxing. They have plenty of fiber, few calories, and hormone-balancing power.
- Design your Keto-Green plate. Typically, my Keto-Green diet adheres to the following ratios: 55–70 percent fats, 5–15 percent carbohydrates, and 20–30 percent protein. On a plate, this means greens and alkalinizing vegetables account for 75 percent of the surface area. Proteins make up a palm-size amount, approximately 4 to 6 ounces. Then imagine a circle in the center of the plate, which equals approximately ¼ cup healthy fats, such as avocados, nuts, or olive oil. For breakfast, feel free to have a Keto-Green Smoothie every morning, one of the smoothies in the recipe section, or any of my Keto-Green breakfast recipes.
- Eat three meals a day with some kind of protein at every meal—vegetarian proteins, eggs, fish, poultry, or grass-fed meat—along with your alkalinizing vegetables. Remember: If you can pick it, peel it, fish it, hunt it, milk it, or grow it, you can eat it on my plan.
- The caveat to my three-meals-a-day rule is when you are doing intermittent prolonged fasts. As you become more practiced at being Keto-Green, you may comfortably be able to have just two meals a day. Personally, I occasionally like to combine my Keto-Green Shake with my lunch meal, but then have nothing else until dinner. Take your time and don't push it, because if you get too aggressive too fast with intermittent fasting, the hunger hormone ghrelin can surge and sabotage even your best intentions.

- Avoid gluten and grains, and avoid refined sugar products, fla-
vorings, colorings, and preservatives altogether. Always build
your diet around Keto-Green whole foods. This is one of the
smartest moves you can make to fix your hormones. I've found
that menopausal and postmenopausal women are energy storers,
so eating grain of any type can pack on the weight, slow us
down, and upset our blood sugar balance. Some occasional rice
and quinoa may be fine for you, but be aware that if you are
struggling at all, you should completely eliminate them.
- Drink approximately half your ideal body weight in ounces of
water each day. But don't drink more than 4 ounces of fluids with
your meals, so that your digestive juices have time to do their
work. My typical recommendation is to drink water up to twenty
minutes before you eat, then have 4 ounces of fluid with your
meal, and wait one to two hours afterward to drink more.
- Continue to take your morning and evening supplements.
- Pay attention to what keeps you satisfied, gives you energy, and
helps you get and stay trim.
- If you find yourself craving something sweet, reach for an alkaline carb fruit like berries with some nuts (see the food list on
pages 311–13). But keep in mind that fruit is a carb, so you don't
want to overdo it. My favorite option is to enjoy a piece of dark
chocolate with a cacao content of 75 percent or more.
- If you are a vegan or vegetarian, follow the swaps listed on
page 77.
- Stay in ketosis. First, restrict your carbohydrate intake (basically,
no bread, cereals, pasta, grains, or other starchy or sugary carbs).
A good guideline is to keep your carbs at around 30 to 40 grams
per day or less.

Also, eat moderate amounts of protein. Women need about 50 to 75
grams of protein daily, which will be reflected in the meal plans—so you
don't have to worry about counting anything.

Increase your fat intake too. Healthy fats help with hormone balance,
keep you feeling satiated, and support hormone production. For a long
time we've been told to be wary of fat, and thus we slashed fat in favor of

carbs. This low-fat movement contributed to the hormonal challenges women face today, I believe.

Good fats to include are avocados, egg yolks, homemade mayo, homemade salad dressings, Hollandaise sauce, nuts, olives, organic grass-fed butter or ghee (on vegetables and meat and in soups). The meal plan figures all this in for you automatically so you can stay in ketosis.

Finally, continue to do Keto-Green fasting overnight, every day, and if you like, monitor your urinary ketones and pH daily, or at least three times a week.

BECOMING KETO-ADAPTED

You'll recall that on day 6 of the Quick Start, you started eating more ketogenic. As you continue with this eating style, your body will gradually become "keto-adapted." Keto-adaptation is the process the body goes through as it switches from using primarily glucose for energy to using primarily fat for energy. Our bodies are always using a mix of fat and glucose for fuel, but in a non-keto-adapted state, the body taps into glucose first. Once you're keto-adapted, your body is basically in a continual state of fat-burning.

As you progress on the twenty-one-day plan, you will begin to feel the positive effects of keto-adaptation. Signs include improved mental concentration and focus, fewer cravings, and even more physical energy. If you have been insulin resistant, your blood pressure and blood sugar usually begin to normalize. By the end of the second to third week of the plan, your body is usually fully adapted to using fat for energy.

Eventually, my Keto-Green plan will become a way of life for you. Your body becomes accustomed to what you feed it, and as you continue along this path, embracing a healthier approach to eating becomes easier. You're awakening your subtle body physiology, honoring what it needs at this stage in your life, and becoming infinitely healthier.

The 21-Day Plan Menus

Here are twenty-one days of breakfasts, lunches, and dinners. The corresponding recipes begin on page 205. Following this plan exactly as written—including using the weekly shopping lists I've also created below—will help you stay on track and see results. But feel free to create your own recipes using the Keto-Green plate guidelines. I also offer some simple alternatives in the sidebar on page 124.

STOCKING YOUR PANTRY

Essential herbs and spices include turmeric, cumin, sea salt, pepper, allspice, garam masala, Mighty Maca Plus, ginger, cardamom, cinnamon, nutmeg, and cayenne pepper. Other things you'll appreciate having in your pantry include Bragg apple cider vinegar, nori sheets, nuts and seeds (including sunflower seeds, sesame seeds, pumpkin seeds, chia seeds, flaxseeds, Brazil nuts [high in selenium], and pili nuts—a type of nut from the Philippines that is high in fat, has zero carbs, and is rich in nutrients). Stock up on healthy fats, including olive oil, coconut oil, MCT oil, avocado oil, and organic ghee and butter from grass-fed cows.

Organize your shopping list to include sections for greens, proteins, veggies, and a few favorite low-carb fruits such as pomegranates, blueberries, and other berries.

Along with your veggies, think avocados, leeks, onions, and garlic. Jicama is a great veggie to add to salads because it's crunchy and very low in carbs.

Choose a selection of fermented and digestive-support foods, including sauerkraut, kimchi, radish, and fresh ginger.

WEEK 1

DAY 1

Breakfast: *Keto-Green Smoothie*
Lunch: *Greek Salad*
Dinner: *Crock-Pot Chicken Soup*

DAY 2

Breakfast: *Keto Omelet Wrap*
Lunch: *Spring Cobb Salad*
Dinner: *Beef Kebobs, Sautéed Beet Greens,* and *Scented Cauliflower Rice*

DAY 3

Breakfast: *Keto-Green Shake*
Lunch: *Spinach and Kale Salad with Bacon and Chicken* drizzled with extra-virgin olive oil or MCT oil and apple cider vinegar
Dinner: *Grilled Salmon with Garlic-Oregano Aioli, Zoodles with Avocado Pesto*

DAY 4

Breakfast: *Keto Chorizo Egg Muffins*
Lunch: *Cleansing Spring Soup*
Dinner: *Flank Steak with Chimichurri Sauce*

DAY 5

Breakfast: *Keto-Green Shake*
Lunch: *Easy Tomato Soup* and *DIY Keto-Green Salad* topped with pumpkin seeds and drizzled with olive oil or MCT oil and apple cider vinegar
Dinner: *Lettuce Tacos*

DAY 6

Breakfast: *Green Eggs and Bacon*

Lunch: *DIY Keto-Green Salad* topped with pumpkin seeds and drizzled with extra-virgin olive oil or MCT oil and apple cider vinegar

Dinner: *Salmon Cakes* with sautéed greens

DAY 7

Breakfast: *Coconut Almond Pancakes*

Lunch: *Avocado Stuffed with Chicken Salad*

Dinner: *Stir-Fry Shrimp with Eggplant and Onions*

Grocery Shopping List for Week 1

In most cases, I do not give quantities. These vary depending on whether you cook for just yourself or for others as well. You should leave a meal feeling satisfied, not stuffed.

Proteins

Bacon
Chicken
Eggs, large, organic, and cage-free
Grass-fed ground beef
Grass-fed steak
Salmon fillets
Shrimp, fresh or frozen
Smoked salmon
Spanish chorizo, pancetta, or pepperoni
Tuna, canned
Turkey breast
Protein powder, 1 canister (a quality protein powder should have fewer than 3 grams sugar and fewer than 10 grams of carbohydrates per serving and contain high-quality protein; see Resources for recommendations)

Dairy*

Cheddar cheese, organic (optional)
Feta and/or goat cheese (optional)
Plain yogurt or kefir (or dairy-free substitute)

Produce

Avocado
Basil

---

* If, after adding in dairy, you get swollen or gain weight, it is best to omit.

Beet greens
Bell pepper, green
Bell pepper, red
Berries
Carrots
Cauliflower
Celery
Chives
Cilantro
Cucumbers
Eggplant
Garlic
Ginger root
Kale
Lemons
Lettuce
Limes
Onion, red
Onion, white or yellow, or shallots
Parsley
Radishes
Scallions
Spinach
Sprouts
Tomatoes
Zucchini

Nuts and Seeds

Almond butter
Almonds
Flaxseeds

Canned Goods and Miscellaneous Ingredients

Almond milk or coconut milk, unsweetened, 1 quart
Chicken, beef, or vegetable broth, 2 quarts
Italian plum tomatoes, 2 cans (28 ounces each)
Unsweetened coconut flakes

WEEK 2

DAY 8
Breakfast: *Keto-Green Smoothie*
Lunch: *DIY Keto-Green Salad* with either salmon, chicken, tuna, or grilled shrimp, drizzled with extra-virgin olive oil or MCT oil and apple cider vinegar
Dinner: *Pan-Roasted Salmon* with *Roasted Spring Veggies*

DAY 9
Breakfast: *Keto-Green Smoothie*
Lunch: *Wild Salmon Salad Wraps*
Dinner: *Chicken* or *Turkey Chili*

DAY 10
Breakfast: *Green Eggs and Bacon*
Lunch: Leftover *Chicken* or *Turkey Chili* and a small green salad drizzled with extra-virgin olive oil or MCT oil and apple cider vinegar
Dinner: *Pan-Roasted Salmon* with *Roasted Spring Veggies*

DAY 11
Breakfast: *Keto-Green Smoothie*
Lunch: *Broccoli Slaw and Egg Salad* over fresh greens with *Easy Tomato Soup*
Dinner: Grilled chicken with *Bacon-Wrapped Asparagus*

DAY 12
Breakfast: *Keto-Coconut Yogurt Berry Bowl*
Lunch: *DIY Keto-Green Salad* (made with spinach) with tuna, drizzled with extra-virgin olive oil or MCT oil and apple cider vinegar
Dinner: *Keto-Green Crock-Pot Lamb and Veggie Stew* with *Sautéed Greens*

DAY 13

Breakfast: *Keto Slow-Cooker Breakfast Casserole*
Lunch: *Thai Coconut Soup*
Dinner: *Coriander-Crusted Ribeye Steaks* with *Zoodles with Avocado Pesto* and sliced tomato

DAY 14

Breakfast: *Coconut Almond Pancakes* with bacon
Lunch: *Oven-Braised Spare Ribs* with *Keto-Green Coleslaw* and sautéed collard greens
Dinner: Leftover *Oven-Braised Spare Ribs*, or turkey burgers with *DIY Keto-Green Salad* drizzled with extra-virgin olive oil or MCT oil and apple cider vinegar

Grocery Shopping List for Week 2

Quantities vary depending on whether you cook for just yourself or for others as well.

Proteins

Bacon
Chicken
Chicken thighs
Eggs, large, organic, and cage-free
Grass-fed steak
Lamb, boneless leg roast
Ribeye steak
Salmon, wild, canned

Produce

Asparagus
Avocados
Baby greens
Bamboo shoots
Basil, fresh
Broccoli slaw mix
Carrots
Celery
Chives
Cilantro
Collard greens
Cucumbers
Dill, fresh
Ginger root
Kaffir lime leaves
Lemongrass stalks
Lemons
Lettuce, romaine and butter

Limes
Mushrooms, crimini
Onions, white or yellow
Parsnips
Poblano peppers
Rosemary, fresh
Scallions
Snap or snow peas
Spinach
Spring vegetables, 1 pound, assorted (carrots, asparagus, baby squash, onions, Brussels sprouts—any veggie suitable for roasting)
Thyme, fresh
Tomatoes
Zucchini

Nuts and Seeds

Almonds
Sunflower seeds

Canned Goods and Miscellaneous Ingredients

Chicken or vegetable broth, 1 quart
Coconut milk, full fat, 8 ounces
Coconut water, 8 ounces
Diced green chiles, small can
Kalamata olives, small jar
Roasted red peppers, 1 jar

WEEK 3

DAY 15

Breakfast: *Keto-Green Smoothie*

Lunch: *Spring Cobb Salad*

Dinner: *Pistachio White Fish* and *Broccoli with Lemon Sauce*

DAY 16

Breakfast: *Keto Chorizo Egg Muffins*

Lunch: *Sesame Seed Chicken Salad*

Dinner: *Spicy Chicken Stir-Fry* (or substitute tempeh or beef for the chicken)

DAY 17

Breakfast: *Keto-Green Smoothie*

Lunch: *Spinach and Kale Salad with Bacon and Chicken,* drizzled with extra-virgin olive oil or MCT oil and apple cider vinegar

Dinner: *Crock-Pot Roast Beef* with sautéed greens

DAY 18

Breakfast: *Green Eggs and Bacon*

Lunch: *DIY Keto-Green Salad* with leftover *Crock-Pot Roast Beef,* drizzled with extra-virgin olive oil or MCT oil and apple cider vinegar

Dinner: *Turkey Tenders with Middle Eastern Spices* and *Keto-Green Coleslaw*

DAY 19

Breakfast: *Keto-Green Smoothie*

Lunch: *Salmon Salad Stuffed Avocado*

Dinner: *Rosemary Seared Lamb Chops* with steamed asparagus

DAY 20

Breakfast: *Eggs Benedict with Smoked Salmon and Spinach*
Lunch: *Chicken Wings with Buffalo Sauce* and *Brussels Sprouts–Kale Salad Bowl*
Dinner: *Cardamom Seared Scallops with Zoodles and Avocado Pesto*

DAY 21

Breakfast: *Keto-Green Smoothie*
Lunch: *Crispy Herb-Roasted Chicken Thighs* with *Mexi-Cauli Rice*
Dinner: *Easy Tomato Soup* or *Bone Broth*

Grocery Shopping List for Week 3

Proteins

Bacon
Beef roast
Chicken breasts
Chicken thighs
Chicken wings
Eggs, large, organic, and cage-free
Lamb chops
Salmon fillets
Salmon, smoked
Scallops
Spanish chorizo or pepperoni
Tempeh, organic
Tilapia or sea bass
Tuna
Turkey breast, roasted, organic
Turkey tenders

Dairy

Cheddar cheese (optional)

Produce

Avocado
Basil, fresh
Bell pepper, yellow
Cabbage, green
Carrots
Cauliflower
Celery
Dill, fresh

Garlic
Kale
Lemons
Lettuce, romaine
Mint, fresh
Onions, red
Onions, white or yellow
Radishes
Snow peas
Spinach, fresh
Spinach, frozen
Sprouts
Tomatoes
Zucchini

Nuts and Seeds

Almonds
Sunflower seeds

Canned Goods and Miscellaneous Ingredients

Italian plum tomatoes, 28-ounce can
Pumpkin, 15-ounce can
Tomato sauce, 15-ounce can
Vegetable broth, low sodium, 1 quart

ALTERNATIVE KETO-GREEN MENU CHOICES

Breakfast Ideas

- 1 cup regular Greek or coconut yogurt with ½ cup strawberries or other berries
- 2 large organic cage-free eggs, any style, with two slices of bacon or sausage patties and side of greens
- 2 large organic cage-free eggs, scrambled with greens
- 1 Keto-Green smoothie (see recipe section for additional smoothie ideas)
- 2 ounces smoked salmon with capers, sliced onions, and tomatoes
- Keto pancakes made with nut flour, served with organic butter and ¼ cup berries
- Tofu veggie scramble
- Eggs Benedict on sliced tomatoes (no bread, of course)

Lunch Ideas

- 4 ounces turkey (white meat) with Dijon mustard, 2 cups raw spinach drizzled with 1 tablespoon healthy oil or MCT oil and a few tablespoons vinegar
- 4 ounces tuna, large mixed green salad with chopped yellow and red bell peppers, drizzled with 2 tablespoons extra-virgin olive oil or MCT oil and lemon juice
- 4 ounces broiled white fish (such as flounder or sole), steamed vegetables with 1 tablespoon melted organic ghee or butter or healthy oil
- 4 ounces shredded chicken mixed with sugar-free mayonnaise and wrapped in lettuce with raw carrots and cucumbers on the side

- 4 ounces stir-fried white fish with 1 cup snow peas, onions, broccoli sprouts, chopped red pepper, and 1 cup cauliflower rice
- Meatless burger or beef or bison burger in lettuce or collard leaf wraps with avocado slices
- Almond butter on celery, bell peppers, and other raw veggies
- Sautéed eggplant with no-sugar marinara sauce
- Black bean soup with a green salad
- Chef's salad with tofu
- Avocado salad (lots of greens topped with avocado and an oil-and-vinegar dressing)
- Tabouli

Dinner Ideas

- 4 ounces broiled red snapper, 1 cup steamed broccoli, and 1 small baked sweet potato with 1 pat organic butter
- 4 ounces London broil, sautéed leeks or onions and mushrooms in wine
- 4 ounces chicken breast with rosemary, 1 cup cauliflower rice, broccoli sautéed in 1 tablespoon olive oil
- Salmon burger patties made with 4 ounces chopped salmon, chopped onions, dill to taste, 1 egg, and ¼ teaspoon sesame seeds, then sautéed in a skillet with 1 tablespoon organic ghee or butter and served with 1 cup steamed cauliflower
- Shrimp sauté: 8 large shrimp sautéed in extra-virgin olive oil and garlic with ½ cup organic tomato sauce (optional after ten-day Quick Start: sprinkled with Parmesan cheese), served over steamed zoodles (zucchini turned into "noodles" using a spiralizer)

- Spaghetti squash or zoodles topped with sautéed veggies and sugar-free marinara sauce
- Vegetarian sloppy joes (ground portobello mushrooms mixed with tomato sauce) and served with a green salad
- Tofurkey meat alternative served with sautéed greens
- Cauliflower rice with stir-fried tofu and various Asian vegetables
- Vegetable stews and soups
- Raw oysters with seaweed salad or broccoli slaw

PART THREE

....

The Keto-Green Lifestyle

Chapter 7

Protect Yourself from Toxic Overload and Hormone Disruptors

You've now been fueling your body with healthy, hormone-fixing, and pH-balancing foods for more than a month. You should be feeling lighter and more energetic, and your perimenopausal or menopausal symptoms should have greatly dissipated. My dearest hope is that your success with this new way of eating will motivate you to keep it up— making Keto-Green eating your way of eating for the foreseeable future.

Remember I said earlier that 75 percent of fixing your hormones has to do with lifestyle changes? That is where we are headed now—lifestyle corrections that will balance your hormones, restore your energy and sensuality, and rejuvenate your body.

Environmental issues can cause hormonal imbalance too—not just exacerbating your perimenopausal or menopausal symptoms but also putting you at higher risks of gynecological diseases (endometriosis, ovarian cysts, infertility, uterine fibroids, cervical dysplasia, fibrocystic breasts, and breast cancer, among others). I've also seen increases in conditions such as fibromyalgia, chronic fatigue syndrome, and thyroid problems, which affect mostly women.

The unfortunate truth is that between the time you leave your house in the morning and when you go to bed at night, you're exposed to hundreds of toxins that can cause hormone havoc, neurological disorders, cancer, and more.

The exposure may start the minute you wake up and jump in the shower. If you have a plastic shower curtain, it contains chemicals that can mess with your hormones.

Oh, and the average shampoo has more than fifteen chemicals in it, many of which disrupt our natural hormones. Antiperspirant packs in more than thirty chemicals. The most injurious is aluminum, which can cause free radical damage to brain cells. After you shower and apply makeup and skin creams, you have already exposed your body to nearly a hundred chemicals.

Commuting to work? Tiny particles from vehicle fumes and other airborne pollutants can trigger respiratory ailments, like pneumonia and asthma, and cause brain inflammation.

In your office, you might be exposed to formaldehyde, which lurks in carpets and furniture made of particleboard. Formaldehyde can irritate your skin and lungs, instigating rashes or aggravating asthma.

Tuna salad for lunch? If it's made with canned white albacore tuna, it may be high in mercury, one of the most toxic substances on earth. That Georgia peach you packed for lunch may be coated with pesticide residues unless it was organically grown.

If you picked up your dry cleaning after work, you've come into contact with perchloroethylene, a chemical widely used in dry-cleaning solution that causes memory loss in humans.

If you need to do a little housework, be aware that many household cleaners are full of strong chemicals—so make sure there's plenty of fresh air circulating while you tidy up.

Overwhelming, isn't it? Over the last hundred years, more than seventy-five thousand types of chemicals have been released into our environment. The majority of these chemicals have never been studied for their cumulative effects on our health and on our children's health.

QUICK TIPS FOR REDUCING
EVERYDAY TOXIN EXPOSURE

- Use an organic-fiber shower curtain instead of plastic.
- Avoid deodorants that contain aluminum. In fact, try making your own deodorant using coconut oil, baking soda, and a little peppermint essential oil.
- If you drive, make sure there's plenty of space between you and other cars; their emissions can get inside your car and accumulate. Or take a less congested route to avoid vehicular pollution. Walking a lot in a city? Stand far from the curb to avoid bus and car fumes.
- If you work in an office where the carpeting or furniture is new, open the windows and door to encourage good ventilation. Demand a high-efficiency particulate air (HEPA) filter. It traps indoor air pollutants such as mold spores, dust, and pollen. Also, decorate your office with houseplants because they help remove toxins from indoor air.
- Tear off plastic covers and air out dry-cleaned items before hanging them in your closet.
- Pick up natural cleaners at a health-food store; they're likely to be toxin-free. Better yet, try white vinegar. It's a simple and inexpensive all-purpose cleaner.

For more toxin-free, natural self-care products, go to the Resources section at the back of this book, or to my website: dranna.com/resources.

In a study spearheaded by the Environmental Working Group in collaboration with Commonweal, researchers at two major laboratories found a total of 287 chemicals and pollutants in umbilical cord blood from ten babies born in August and September 2004 in U.S. hospitals.

Of those 287 chemicals, it is known that 180 cause cancer in humans or animals, 217 are toxic to the brain and nervous system, and 208 cause birth defects or abnormal development in animal tests. The dangers of pre- or postnatal exposure to this complex mixture of carcinogens, developmental toxins, and neurotoxins have never been studied.

What we do know is that many chemicals and pollutants are hormone disruptors. Technically, a hormone disruptor is any substance that alters or mimics normal hormone levels or function in the body. Many man-made chemicals, for example, can upset the normal activity of estrogens, androgens, thyroid, and other hormones. They latch on to hormone receptors on cells and activate them, blocking normal hormonal action or interfering with proteins that regulate the activity of hormones. They are hard for the body to break down and eliminate. Sadly, our bodies are becoming inundated with them. Further, they invade your neuroendocrine system, where they can cause estrogen dominance, reduced libido, sexual dysfunction, mood swings, inflammation, immune disorders, cancer, metabolic syndrome, and more.

So what should we do about these toxins? Well, we can't force giant chemical companies to stop making them, but we can try to vote with our dollars by doing our very best to stop buying plastics, drugs, and chemicals, and we can take personal action to clean up our bodies. It can be done.

A patient of mine named Christy is proof. She came to me six years after having been aggressively treated with chemotherapy, radiation, and bilateral mastectomy for a very serious form of breast cancer diagnosed at age thirty-nine.

Now forty-five, Christy was really struggling. She was moody, felt fatigued, and complained of hot flashes that were relentless and a persistent brain fog. All of her hormones were low, especially vitamin D. Her body was not properly detoxifying estrogen, and she had very low levels of omega-3 fats. There was a lot of inflammation going on in her body, and heavy metal testing showed that she had toxic lead exposure.

In talking with Christy I learned that her exposure over the years to noxious chemicals had been intense. As a child, Christy had been on antibiotics for long stretches of time due to upper respiratory illnesses. So here was my first clue. Antibiotics can cause gut bacteria imbalances that can last for years because they destroy not just the bad bacteria but the good bacteria too, which is our first line of defense and supports a healthy immune system and healthy estrogen detoxification.

Christy also grew up in a farming community where crops were heavily sprayed with pesticides, which are known hormone disruptors. As a young adult, she worked in a factory that had a lot of formaldehyde in and on the premises. I learned she had had severe gastrointestinal symptoms and irritable bowel syndrome the entire time she was employed there. Additionally, she had been on birth control pills for many years. Birth control pills do cause hormone disruption. They contain synthetic progestins and utilize the body's natural minerals and B vitamins for metabolism, further disrupting gut microbes and bringing on hormone havoc.

I can't ever know for sure if any or all of these factors contributed to Christy's cancer diagnosis at such a young age, but I didn't want to wait another day to help her detoxify and get healthy again.

Together, Christy and I worked on improving her estrogen metabolism through detoxification, nutrition, supplementation, and reduced exposure to environmental toxins. Supplements that I added were diindolylmethane (DIM, a compound found in cruciferous vegetables and used for hormone balance), vitamins E, C, and D, omega-3s, methylated B vitamins, Mighty Maca Plus (my green superfood drink), a detoxification support supplement, and ultra-low-dose bioidentical hormone therapy that included estriol, estradiol, progesterone, testosterone, and DHEA.

After going Keto-Green for a month, Christy reported feeling "Ninety percent better!" Today she is in her midfifties and doing beautifully—no recurrence of breast cancer, thank God. I share her powerful story to let you know that we have a lot of control over hormone disruptors and other toxins and the quality of our lives. Like Christy, you can be empowered to heal and to live your best quality of life. As she puts it, "There is no better investment than your health."

As my emphasis throughout this book has certainly made clear, investing in your health starts with your food! Shopping and eating the Keto-Green way will ensure that you steer clear of the toxic chemicals too often used in food production, but here is a rundown of other strategies for protecting yourself against toxins and chemicals in your food supply.

- Buy organic fruits and vegetables grown without pesticides, herbicides, synthetic fertilizer, or hormones. If you buy conventional produce, familiarize yourself with the Clean 15 and the Dirty Dozen, put together by the Environmental Working Group. (See the latest list in the following box.)
- Purchase organic, free-range, grass-fed, hormone-free meats, eggs, and other animal products.
- Eat fish low in mercury, including sardines, anchovies, and wild-caught salmon. Most other seafood fits this bill, but there are exceptions: albacore tuna, swordfish, shark, king mackerel, red snapper, orange roughy, moonfish, bass, marlin, and trout. If you eat any of these fish, limit your servings to once a week.
- Visit the Environmental Working Group's website, ewg.org, for a list of foods lowest in pesticides and fish lowest in mercury.
- Grilling your meat on high heat, to the point where you cause charring, releases heterocyclic amines (HCAs). High intake levels are linked to an increased risk of pancreatic, colorectal, and stomach cancer. Marinating the meat and cooking it at medium or low temperatures will drastically cut HCA formation. So will serving your meat with a side of cabbage, which limits the creation of these chemicals by 17 to 20 percent, says a 2014 study published in *Food Chemistry*.
- As I explained in Chapter 4, emphasize the cruciferous family of veggies (broccoli, broccoli sprouts, cauliflower, cabbage, and so forth), as well as garlic, onions, and leeks. These foods enhance detoxification due to their high content of the sulfur-containing amino acids cysteine and methionine. They also contain the antioxidants DIM and indole-3-carbinol (I3C), which play a part in fighting off certain cancer-causing substances in the body. Their extra fiber helps escort pseudo-estrogens from the body.
- Stay alkaline. Eat more vegetables that are high in alkalizing minerals, such as potassium, magnesium, and calcium. Avocados, unsweetened cocoa powder, and dried herbs such as dill,

basil, oregano, turmeric, and saffron are rich in potassium (forgo the bananas and the beans because they're high in starch). Green leafy vegetables are packed with magnesium, methylators, and more. Broccoli, sea vegetables, and collard greens are high in calcium. Don't forget your bone or alkaline broth for a mineral boost. An alkaline diet helps greatly to remove toxins, reduce inflammation, and enhance overall health and energy.

- Drink more fluids, especially water. Staying well hydrated daily flushes toxins from your body. Filtered water is best. You may have heard about the catastrophic contamination of the water supply in Flint, Michigan, which had increased levels of lead in the drinking water. This was a result of improper water treatment and water pipe corrosion. High lead is known to increase mental illness, ADD, irrational behavior, and anger, and children are especially vulnerable. Not coincidentally, Flint has been one of the most violent cities in the United States. Certainly toxins play a role in this. I feel strongly that physiology guides behavior. Bottom line: filter your water!

- Get sweaty. Perspiration—a mix of water, salt, and waste—is a natural detoxifying system. So exercise at high intensity (I like hot yoga for detoxifying) or sit in a steam room or sauna. Infrared saunas are particularly helpful because they have been shown in studies to do an excellent job of releasing toxins from the body. See the Resources section for more information on detoxifying products.

The Dirty Dozen

According to the Environmental Working Group, these foods are heavily sprayed with pesticides and have pesticide residues on them. It is best to purchase organic versions of these fruits and vegetables.

1. Strawberries
2. Spinach

3. Nectarines
4. Apples

5. Grapes
6. Peaches
7. Cherries
8. Pears

9. Tomatoes
10. Celery
11. Potatoes
12. Bell peppers

The Clean 15

Although organic produce is best, it is safe to purchase conventionally grown versions of these fruits and vegetables, as these foods have very little pesticide residue on them or in them. Still, wash thoroughly.

1. Avocados
2. Sweet corn
3. Pineapples
4. Cabbages
5. Onions
6. Sweet peas
7. Papayas
8. Asparagus

9. Mangoes
10. Eggplant
11. Honeydew melon
12. Kiwi
13. Cantaloupe
14. Cauliflower*
15. Broccoli*

* I still prefer that you always buy organic versions of these two vegetables because of their detoxifying powers, breast-cancer-protective qualities, and nutrient density.

Navigating Your Food Supply

Above and beyond the general guidelines above, here is my advice for reducing your exposure to pesticides, chemicals, and other toxins in your environment and food supply.

GMOs

Genetically modified organisms (GMOs) are created in labs, using a cut-and-paste procedure for altering DNA. Genetic engineers take genes from one living thing (say, a bacterium) and insert them into the DNA of another living thing (for example, a type of corn) to endow it with new traits (such as pest resistance).

Today, genetically modified ingredients are found in at least 75 percent of all non-organic U.S. processed foods, including in many products labeled as "natural" or "all natural." But are they good for us? Our government says GMOs are no biggie, yet the European Union, Australia, and Japan have restricted or banned them. Based on animal research, the American Academy of Environmental Medicine (AAEM), an international organization of physicians, has stated that there are serious health problems linked to eating genetically modified foods, such as infertility, immune system problems, accelerated aging, insulin problems, cholesterol regulation, gut problems, and organ damage.

Protect yourself:
- Choose organic food. This is an easy way to steer clear of GMOs and suspected and unsuspected risks that may come with them. Organic farmers are not allowed to plant genetically modified seeds.
- Buy local. Small farmers often employ organic practices, including shunning GMOs.
- Stay away from packaged foods as much as possible, and avoid vegetable oils like soybean and canola oils—most of which are made from genetically modified crops. Most unprocessed whole foods are GMO-free. And the fact that whole foods are good for you is, happily, not up for debate.
- If you buy any packaged or processed foods, look for a Non-GMO Project Verified label, which means the product has undergone a rigorous review and testing process.
- When eating out, understand that Mexican cuisine (which uses lots of corn) and Asian cuisine (which uses lots of soy) tend to have a lot of genetically modified ingredients. By contrast, Greek, Italian, and Middle Eastern restaurants most likely use 100 percent olive oil and are thus much better choices for avoiding GMO meals. Find out what a restaurant uses; ask the server before you order!

BPA and Phthalates

Bisphenol A (BPA) is a chemical found in plastics used to make compact discs, plastic bottles, the lining of metal food cans, and dental sealants. It leaches out of plastics into food and the environment. BPA stimulates estrogen receptors and has been linked to breast cancer.

Phthalates are added to plastic products to make them strong, yet soft and pliable. They are also used in carpet backing, paints, glues, insect repellants, hair spray, and nail polish. Phthalates are hormone disruptors and can suppress ovulation and normal estrogen production, cause premature breast development in young girls, and contribute to polycystic ovary syndrome (PCOS), according to many studies performed over the last ten to fifteen years.

Protect yourself:
- Avoid plastic products whenever you can. If you do purchase something packaged in plastic, transfer it to a glass container.
- Store your food in glass or ceramic containers, rather than in plastic.
- Do not heat or microwave food in plastic containers or with plastic wrap over the top. (Another reason to avoid microwaves as much as possible: they can decrease the antioxidant content of foods.)
- Buy your condiments in glass containers instead of plastic.
- If you buy canned food, look for "BPA-free" on labels.
- Use an organic-fiber shower curtain instead of plastic.
- Use cloth bags for carrying home groceries instead of plastic bags.
- Avoid water, soft drinks, and baby formula sold in polycarbonate (clear plastic) bottles. If possible, use only glass bottles.
- Know your local farmers and what they use on their produce. Try growing your own; a lot can be grown in small areas and planters.
- Ask for your receipt to be emailed instead of printed. Printed receipts contain toxins (BPA), so it's best not to handle them.
- Forgo plastic straws and remove plastic lids from that to-go coffee, or use a reusable stainless steel cup or mug.

Dioxins

Dioxins are a by-product from the production of chlorine-containing products like pesticides, wood preservatives, and the bleaching of paper. They can linger in the environment for years and pile up in the food chain. They diminish thyroid hormones and testosterone, and mimic estrogen in the body. They are also linked to endometriosis as well as to increased rates of stillbirth.

Protect yourself:
- Eat thyroid-protective foods such as natural iodine-containing foods, including sea vegetables (nori, hijiki, dulse, and kelp) and low-carb kelp noodles. Enjoy a wide variety of low-mercury fish a few times a week. My other favorite thyroid-supporting foods are oysters and Brazil nuts. I highly recommend two Brazil nuts daily, which will provide approximately 200 micrograms of selenium, a mineral that supports the thyroid, brain, and metabolism.
- Ease off your use of bleached paper products. Unbleached coffee filters, for example, are available from several companies, as are reusable filters.
- Choose earth-friendly clothes made of natural fibers for your wardrobe.
- Avoid bedding and clothes treated with flame retardants.
- When remodeling, avoid vinyl flooring. It may release harmful chemicals such as phthalates and dioxin, according to the Healthy Building Network. Install tile, bamboo, or solid wood flooring, if possible.

Pesticides

Dangerous chemicals such as DDT have been banned in this country for many years, but their residues still persist in the environment. DDT was an insecticide heavily used in agriculture and for killing mosquitoes. It is an estrogen disruptor and has harmful effects on memory and learning. In general, pesticides have been linked to infertility, spontaneous abortion, and breast cancer, according to reports in *Fertility and Sterility, BCERF,* and other scientific journals.

Today, our industrial food supply is mostly grown with a pesticide called glyphosate, the active ingredient in the weed killer called Roundup. Glyphosate is a very scary pesticide. It acts as an antibiotic that can kill bacteria, and emerging scientific evidence suggests that it may lead to a harmful imbalance in bacteria in soil and in the human gut. Researchers also believe it may act as a hormone disruptor.

Glyphosate has been associated with a host of health issues such as kidney disease, liver disease, reproductive problems, neurological diseases, and birth defects. The link between glyphosate and cancer is particularly unsettling. In 2015, the International Agency for Research on Cancer (IARC), part of the World Health Organization, declared glyphosate a "probable human carcinogen."

Protect yourself:
- Steer clear of glyphosate-sprayed food by seeking out products that bear the USDA Organic label.
- Avoid pesticides as much as possible. Instead, practice healthier pest management by sealing cracks, fixing leaks, and cleaning up food residues. Where infestations require treatment, follow least-toxic extermination practices.
- Use organic pesticides. Boric acid is widely available. Neem leaves and oil come from a tree native to India and are well known for their ability to repel insects. Sprinkle diatomaceous earth around the outside of your home's foundation. Diatomaceous earth is a substance made of crushed fossils from underwater marine life that is deadly to insects but harmless to humans, but please note, inhalation should be avoided.
- Remove your shoes when entering the house to prevent tracking fertilizer or pesticide residues into the house.
- Grow insect-repelling plants such as basil, chives, mint, and marigolds.

Formaldehyde

Formaldehyde is a chemical that was used in insulation in the 1970s. But its fumes caused depression, fatigue, poor memory, headaches, asthma, cough, skin rashes, and much more. Formaldehyde is no longer found in insulation, but it is present in many products we use daily: shampoo, conditioners, cosmetics, cleaning supplies, carpet, paper products, plastics, and more. It has been linked to reduced fertility, spontaneous abortion, endometriosis, and cancer.

Protect yourself:
- Look for formaldehyde-free products; check labels.
- Don't purchase sheets that say "easy-care" or "permanent press" on the label; they are commonly treated with formaldehyde. Consider untreated organic cotton sheets.
- If you own particleboard or plywood furniture, consider coating it with AFM's SafeCoat Safe Seal, a sealant with a very tight molecular structure that prevents outgassing of formaldehyde.
- Do not use e-cigarettes. Existing research suggests that dripping liquid nicotine directly onto the devices' atomizers can expose users to formaldehyde in the vapors.
- Avoid candles made with paraffin, a petroleum-derived wax that the EPA has found can emit trace amounts of chemicals like toluene and formaldehyde. Instead, burn candles made from beeswax and scented with essential oils. These do not emit toxins.
- Make sure your home and work environments are properly ventilated—and don't forget to use HEPA filters and air-purifying houseplants.

Heavy Metals

Although trace amounts of some metals such as copper, iron, and iodine are necessary for good health, in excessive amounts, metals such as arsenic, cadmium, mercury, and lead have been found to stimulate estrogen receptors and are therefore considered hormone disruptors. Sources of arsenic include some brands of rice, some seafood, and some well water. Cadmium is found in cigarettes and some yellow paint. Mercury is mostly in larger fish and old amalgam dental fillings. Lead is a component of air pollution, paint and dyes, and ceramic glazes, among other sources.

Various heavy metals are linked to many women's health conditions. Exposure to cadmium, mercury, manganese, lead, and arsenic may limit fertility. Low to moderate lead exposures may increase the risk for spontaneous abortion.

I often test for heavy metals and minerals in my patients with difficult diagnoses or medical conditions such as autoimmune diseases, Hashimoto's disease, cancer, endometriosis, memory issues, and infertility. I nearly always find elevated levels.

Protect yourself:
- Supplement with natural chelators. Chelators bind with toxic heavy metals so they can be excreted. Vitamin C is a potent one. Researchers at the University of Texas Medical Branch at Galveston found that adult smokers who took 1,000 milligrams daily of vitamin C dramatically lowered lead levels in their blood within one week.
- Eat chelating foods. High-sulfur foods such as ginger, garlic, cilantro, onions, broccoli sprouts, and eggs help scavenge and safely remove from the body any toxic metals that they come in contact with. Curcumin reduces the toxic injury to the liver induced by arsenic, cadmium, chromium, copper, lead, and mercury, according to research published in *Food and Chemical Toxicology* in 2014. And sesame oil is potently beneficial for treating lead- and iron-induced liver and kidney toxicity, says a 2014 report in *Journal of Parenteral and Enteral Nutrition*. Clearly, nutritious food goes a long way toward abating the toxic effects of heavy metals.
- Talk to your dentist about safely removing mercury fillings and replacing them with nontoxic options. Alternatively, find a holistic dentist who takes a more integrative approach. If you choose to remove amalgam fillings, I recommend that you:

Detox first

Increase your vitamin C to 4,000 IU daily

Use a probiotic daily

Increase intake of the omega-3s EPA and DHA to 3,000 to 4,000 mg
daily

Additional supplements that I would recommend adding are Pura
Detox support (2 capsules twice daily), liposomal glutathione, Mighty
Maca Plus, and NAC.

Parabens and Other Cosmetic Chemicals

Parabens are used as preservatives in thousands of cosmetics, foods, and
pharmaceutical products, including bioidentical hormone creams.
Parabens are known hormone disruptors. A 2004 study published in the
Journal of Applied Toxicology found a high concentration of parabens in
human breast tumors.

Protect yourself:
- Find products labeled paraben-free and phthalate-free, but always check ingredients. Look out for products containing hard-
  to-pronounce chemicals like methylparaben, ethylparaben, and
  butylparaben as well as dicyclohexyl phthalate (DCP), diisononyl
  phthalate (DINP), and di-n-propyl phthalate (DPP).
- Switch to natural/organic cosmetics and grooming products. Or
  try making your own cosmetics and skin care products from
  natural sources. It's easy to do, and there are many recipes on the
  Internet.
- Wear a hat and tightly woven fabrics for sun protection. Sunscreens, even alternative ones, can contain chemicals such as cy-
  closiloxane, a hormone disruptor. Choose your sunscreen wisely.
- Avoid hand sanitizers. These products contain two hormone-
  disrupting chemicals: triclosan and triclocarban. They're marketed as germ fighters, but don't work much better than soap

and water, according to the Centers for Disease Control and Prevention. In fact, their use can disrupt your natural bacterial defense.

- Go to the Environmental Working Group's website, ewg.org, or to goodguide.com for information on chemicals in various cosmetics.

Household Chemicals

Most of us consider our homes safe havens from what seems an increasingly toxic world. Oh, if only! Unfortunately, they are often filled with products and chemicals that may threaten health. And much of the time we're not even aware of it. One study published in *Environmental Health Perspectives* indicated that consumers who use fragranced products (perfume, air fresheners, dryer sheets) and sunscreens expose themselves to an array of hormone disruptors that are potentially toxic.

Disinfectants are a nice idea, but they contain phenol and cresol, which can cause diarrhea, fainting, dizziness, and kidney and liver damage. Furniture and floor polishes are formulated with a nasty chemical called nitrobenzene, which if inhaled can irritate your lungs and if ingested can cause poisoning and death. The chemical has also been associated with cancer and birth defects.

Protect yourself:
- Purchase the least harmful household cleaners available. Look for the words "biodegradable" and "nontoxic" on the label.
- Clean the way your grandmother did. Stick with water, baking soda, and white vinegar. Or make your own natural cleaners; you can find many great recipes on the Internet. You can make a glass cleaner, for example, by mixing 1 tablespoon lemon juice in 1 quart of water. Spray on and wipe dry. A simple mixture of baking soda or vinegar, scrubbed on with a toilet brush, makes a great toilet cleaner. You can polish furniture with 1 tablespoon lemon juice in 1 pint mineral or vegetable oil.

- Disinfect germy spots like toilet handles and doorknobs with vinegar or hydrogen peroxide. Or add plain old liquid dish soap to a bucketful of hot water and start scrubbing away the nasties.
- Switch to natural cleaning products. I list brands I like in the Resources section.
- Use an alkalinizing laundry water–filtration system. I have one and typically only wash my laundry with a little bit of boric acid or a natural cleaner.

The issues related to toxins may seem overwhelming, but pause with me a moment and take a deep breath. Yes, it is disheartening to hear about all the toxic and potentially toxic substances that we have been exposed to and which affect us and future generations.

Although you can't completely avoid them, you can limit your exposure to hormone disruptors and other environmental contaminants, step by step. Start making the shifts I suggest, but do it now. If you apply even a few of these strategies, you'll greatly minimize the effects of toxins on your body. Controlling your exposure to hormone-disrupting compounds begins simply with choices made at home and at the store. You can do it, and your ongoing health is well worth the effort.

Chapter 8

Stop Stress from Stressing You Out

As much as any environmental toxin, chronic stress can be a hormone disruptor too. But as with chemicals and pesticides, there are things you can do to reduce your exposure to chronic stress—as well as mitigate your response to it. I know this personally all too well.

On March 12, 2006—a few weeks before Easter—we had friends over for lunch after church, and everyone was enjoying the beautiful day. Nothing about the day indicated that my life was moments away from changing forever.

I can remember the sermon from church that day as well. The priest was talking about Abraham, who was called from God to sacrifice his son Isaac, and I thought, *What a crazy old man. Our children are so, so precious.*

That tragic day, my children were playing together inside, and I slipped away to use the bathroom. When I came out, my eighteen-month-old son, Garrett, was not with his sisters. I immediately knew something was very terribly wrong.

What followed next was beyond my worst nightmare, playing out in slow motion. I looked out the side door, then the back door, and then I found him. Somehow he had managed to get outside without triggering the door alarms and had fallen into our swimming pool. I raced to the pool, pulled him out of the water, and started mouth-to-mouth resuscitation right away. My nine-year-old daughter called an ambulance, and a neighbor who had heard my screams came to help.

Garrett had a pulse and paramedics prepared to race him to our small local hospital, but they refused to let me ride in the ambulance with my baby, despite my desperate protest. I know they too were doing all they could, but everything that could go wrong did go wrong. For instance, the breathing tube could not be inserted, and the ambulance was delayed in finding the entrance to the emergency room because it had recently been moved to the opposite side of the hospital. Garrett died at the hospital.

The next days are still a blur to me; I was in a trance of sorts. We refused to let our baby go—I even carried him into his funeral. Amid our friends, our community, and complete compassionate strangers, I handed him to our priest. The world as we knew it had come to an end.

My heart was irrevocably shattered for my son and for my family, my daughters and my husband. I faced and battled all the demons of losing a child—shame, fear, guilt, and blame, of myself and others. The emotional trauma was devastating. Nothing in our lives was ever ordinary again. Years have passed now, but I cry as I write this and there are still days where grief washes over me.

If you have endured grief and loss, it is important to not compare your experience with mine. That only minimizes it. All of our experiences, no matter how different, are real, and the emotional depth that we feel is ours to honor.

I can step away now and intellectualize from a medical perspective what trauma and grief do to us. There are physical consequences, for sure. I went through this myself. One of the earliest signs had to do with my breast milk. I had been breastfeeding Garrett every day of his life, and after the accident, not another drop of milk flowed from my breasts.

My heart physically ached in my chest. The heart feels tragedy. It is an endocrine organ that also has receptors for and produces oxytocin, the love and connection hormone. Agony depletes oxytocin. My body ached too. It hurt to put my feet on the floor in the morning.

My periods became irregular. Then they stopped altogether, because I developed premature ovarian failure and was told I was irreversibly in early menopause, which also meant I would not be able to have any more children, something we had planned for before losing Garrett.

I had trouble sleeping, not to mention checking on my sleeping children once, twice, even three times a night.

Tragedy affects relationships. I knew that statistics show that more than 70 percent of married couples divorce after the loss of a child. We were determined not to be part of that statistic. But we were struggling.

Of course, there were emotional effects too. I was depressed. The world around me sometimes felt foggy, and I struggled to make sense of even the simplest things. Life had lost all its color because I was overcome with grief. Although I wanted to escape my life, I held my family close and stayed strong for them. I wanted to give them a better example of how to handle adversity, stand up, and keep moving forward.

I needed some privacy to grieve, but I also needed to keep the earth moving under my feet. I would jokingly say that I had to travel around the world to learn that everywhere you go, there you are!

And so we decided to take some time as a family away from the place with which we associated so much sadness. I left my practice in the good hands of a trusted colleague, Dr. Deborah Shepherd. She enabled us to go on a healing journey. Travel for me has always been my meditation and a large part of my education, so I reasoned that traveling, experiencing indigenous cultures, and exposing our daughters to the world might help us. I'd arranged home exchanges and visits with family and friends around the world.

As I traveled, I learned native healing therapies. I asked what people did to heal fertility, to heal from grieving, and to apply spiritual and physical connections. I studied their foods, and I spoke with some of the most intuitive, as well as some of the leading physicians around the world. Our journey took me to Native American shamans and then into South America, the mountains of Peru and the Andes, which was where I learned about maca and the herb *una de gato*, or cat's claw. From there, we went to Brazil and Argentina, and then to New Zealand and Australia, and several countries in Asia, the Middle East, and then Europe. I homeschooled my children along the way—a sign that I was partly insane!

Our time away and my exposure to other healing modalities was indeed restorative. As I began to heal physically and emotionally, I did conceive again. It happened more than a year after Garrett had passed away and after I was told I was infertile and in early menopause. We learned the happy news in Israel—I couldn't help but feel we'd experienced a kind of holy miracle!

After coming home, pregnant and grateful, I returned to my practice in full swing and tried to resume life as it had been. I poured myself into my work, bringing much of what I learned from our world journey and world medicine into my holistic practice. But it's clear to me now that I suffered post-traumatic stress disorder (PTSD) for a long time after our return. I didn't really understand it. But I knew I felt like a train going downhill with no brakes—out of control and scared a lot of the time. And, sadly, my marriage was falling apart—we were becoming the statistic we swore we would evade. Three years later, we divorced.

Stress comes in all shapes and sizes—we worry about our children, our parents, our finances, our health, our jobs. We are exposed to stressful news, situations, and people on a daily basis, and the combined load of it all produces chronic stress, which can, as the details of my own personal story show, affect the quality of our lives in so many ways. But it doesn't have to be that way. When I began devoting my life to hormone balance, I was stunned at the lack of information and understanding about the relationship between stress and hormone levels. My own trauma forced me to understand it, piece together its puzzle, and make sense of it so that I could ultimately help my clients heal. I know personally and professionally that each of us can take control over the amount of stress in our lives and stop its assault on our hormones, health, and relationships. In time, you can—as I did—become more resilient and better equipped to heal from stress.

Stress, You, and Your Hormones

Located atop the kidneys, the adrenal glands quietly produce more than fifty hormones that are necessary for your survival. Stress—whether perceived or real—can lead to their overproduction and alter their balance in significant ways.

In response to stress, a hormonal cascade of events occurs in the body, leading to the release of cortisol in the bloodstream, which in turn allows your body to quickly react to the stress you are experiencing.

Cortisol is actually manufactured from another hormone called pregnenolone. Pregnenolone is commonly called the "mother hormone" because in addition to cortisol, it is the hormone from which estrogen, progesterone, testosterone, and DHEA are also derived. Pregnenolone therefore plays a major role in the hormonal symphony in your body.

Under stress, though, the body preferentially calls on pregnenolone to make cortisol in order to handle the pressure you are experiencing. But when pregnenolone is pressed into service to produce cortisol, very little estrogen, DHEA, and testosterone are made. Daily, unresolved stress therefore jeopardizes your normal hormone production.

Cortisol is not inherently a good or bad hormone. It just does what it was designed to do, which is to help the body to respond to stress, a challenge, or a threat. It has a natural circadian rhythm that is vital for quality of life. Its production peaks in the morning—which wakes you up and gets you out of bed, hastening an energetic day. Then it goes down in the evening, signaling bedtime, and normally stays low during sleep.

Cortisol is also a natural anti-inflammatory. Too much cortisol is bad. Too little cortisol is even worse. Cortisol in perfect balance with other hormones optimizes health.

Some stress can be good, even necessary for life. It helps keep us fit, alert, and ready for challenges. But it is bad when relentless. The adrenal glands keep on responding with no chance to normalize, resulting in excess cortisol levels in the blood. This can cause high blood sugar, insulin resistance, high blood pressure, metabolic syndrome, immune system suppression and autoimmune disorders, protein catabolism (the body breaks down protein from its own muscles for energy), osteoporosis, behavioral issues, insomnia, and even hypothyroidism.

Persistent stress can also turn the natural circadian rhythm upside down, causing a restless energy at night and a low during the day (what we call the "tired and wired" sensation). Low cortisol all day creates a devastating condition called hypocortisolism, otherwise known as adrenal fatigue. It is common in people with PTSD, chronic fatigue, adverse childhood experiences such as abuse, and fibromyalgia. It feels like burnout.

ADRENAL BURNOUT

The adrenal glands don't actually give out, but through a feedback system, part of your brain, the paraventricular nucleus of the hypothalamus, sometimes is told to back off and stop producing corticotrophin-releasing factor because, in essence, too much cortisol has been frying our system, specifically the mitochondria—the energy powerhouses of our cells. This is why adrenal fatigue is so complex and hard to treat.

Why is this a big deal?

Because the adrenal glands are part of the HPA-G axis. Its component glands—the hypothalamus, the pituitary, and the adrenals—communicate among one another and with the sex glands or gonads (ovaries or testes) to make sure our hormones are balanced. If one of these organs in the HPA-G axis (such as the adrenal glands) gets imbalanced, this can disrupt the delicate dance of hormones that keep you feeling healthy, happy, and sexy.

Unfortunately, today's modern lifestyle is highly stressful, and it seems almost as though it was designed to create hormone imbalance. We spend our days indoors doing sedentary work. Our families are separated for most of the day and even in some cases, much longer. We fill our brains with stressful images from TV, computers, tablets, and phones. We can't wind down, and we feel like we have to keep performing. It's no wonder that so many visits to primary care physicians are for stress-related complaints.

PTSD AND WOMEN

If "post-traumatic stress disorder" makes you think of battle-scarred soldiers returning from war, you're not alone. Until the turn of the millennium, most doctors thought of PTSD as battle fatigue too. But today we know you don't have to fight in military combat to develop it. Acknowledged triggers of PTSD include domestic violence, child abuse, adverse childhood experiences, sexual assault, a serious traffic accident, a serious illness or injury, being the victim of a crime, suffering natural or man-made disaster, and many other things outside the range of normal human experience. Any of these experiences can alter stress hormones and, therefore, behavior.

Women have been hit hard by PTSD. According to the National Center for PTSD, about 10 of every 100 (or 10 percent) of women develop PTSD sometime in their lives, compared with about 4 of every 100 (or 4 percent) of men.

Although PTSD has different degrees of severity, it mobilizes cortisol. Some trauma is so disturbing—especially sexual trauma in women—that the cortisol stress response does not turn off. In such cases, levels of cortisol and other normally protective stress hormones become imbalanced and cease their protective power. This imbalance begins to usher in heart disease, fatigue, behavioral problems, depression, anxiety, and more.

Chronic stress also depletes the hormones progesterone and pregnenolone, which protect the female brain and support memory and mood. This can lead to a very difficult period around menopause, when progesterone levels are already rapidly dropping.

Additionally, in women with PTSD there is a significant decrease in the conversion of progesterone into allopregnenolone. Allopregnenolone is the hormone that increases levels of GABA, the neurotransmitter that makes us feel good, calm, and *ahh*.

Another huge factor in a woman's response to stress is oxytocin. Under short-term stress, oxytocin levels aren't actually disrupted. The presence of that hormone can make you feel calmer, less afraid, and more social. But with unrelenting stress, chronically elevated levels of cortisol decrease oxytocin production, and you start feeling disconnected from everyone and everything. And when our circadian circuitry is further disrupted—when we have chronic low cortisol with chronic low oxytocin—this emotional disconnect is worsened.

This is exactly what happened to me in the years following my son's death—I kind of checked out and detached from many around me. Ultimately, however, I came to understand the relationship between cortisol and oxytocin, and what to do about it. For me and so many of my clients, it was a powerful revelation just to understand how this physiologic disruption causes us to feel disconnected, alone, and burned out, no longer loving the things and activities and, most important, the people we once did. Knowing that there is a physiological reason for feeling this way is amazingly validating.

Stress Solutions

The good news in all this is that we can reset and restore our optimal physiology, empowering us in mind, body, and spirit. There are simple strategies that can reduce stress and calm your mind.

Stress management will look different for you than it does for me. My personal favorite strategies are taking a walk, going to a yoga or boxing class, and taking a mineral bath with essential oils. I also read something inspirational, such as a devotional, and I meditate too. To be honest, quieting my mind and meditating are challenging for me, but I've found a good resource in a product called the Muse headband. It senses activity in the frontal cortex of the brain (the region responsible for impulse control, problem solving, and judgment) and gives you biofeedback, a treatment technique that trains you to improve your health by using signals from your own body.

The key is to incorporate activities *you* love into your daily routine. Maybe painting or sculpting relaxes you—or exercising, being in nature, reading a great book, or just kicking back and watching your favorite TV shows. In the long run, developing your own techniques will serve you well in managing your physical, mental, and emotional health. Here are some other specific activities to consider in order to create resilience and defend yourself against stress and the hormonal imbalances it creates.

Stay Nutritionally Alkaline

Keeping our stress levels in check starts with nourishing our bodies with foods that heal. Following my Keto-Green diet is the first, most basic step. Enjoying more alkaline foods (especially green plants) helps to normalize cortisol, supports your adrenal glands and gut bacterial health, and improves your natural progesterone levels. Eating healthy fats, especially naturally sourced DHA—which can be found in foods like fish and flaxseeds—is also hormone-healing.

Then, as this book emphasizes throughout, you can get into ketosis. This targets insulin and makes your body more insulin-sensitive. As a result, you'll become more hormone-balanced, with fewer stress-provoking symptoms such as hot flashes, weight gain, and foggy thinking. Ketosis also prevents fluctuations in blood sugar, which place unnecessary strain on adrenal function and are a common cause of excess cortisol production.

Consider Extra Supplements

On page 81, I provide a rundown of the daily supplements I recommend to my patients who are on the Keto-Green Diet: a daily multivitamin, omega-3 fatty acids (via fish oil), vitamin C, magnesium, a probiotic, a liver detoxifier (if your self-test determined you need one), fiber, and maca. If you've been diagnosed with adrenal fatigue or exhaustion, however, you may need to take a few more.

In some cases of adrenal fatigue, your doctor may prescribe cortisol supplements. These can be a helpful *temporary* measure to help reset or reinvigorate your adrenal glands, allowing them to begin secreting cortisol again by themselves. However, long-term cortisol use can shut down the adrenals completely, which has a harmful effect on hormonal balance in general.

Vitamins and minerals. A supplement with high-quality bioavailable B vitamins is essential, including methylated folate, B6, B12, and B5. Extra B vitamins are needed for adrenal support above and beyond what you find in a typical multivitamin formula.

Zinc is a good mineral to supplement if you are under a lot of stress. An active component in more than eighty identified jobs in the body, zinc plays a vital role in many biological processes. Chronic stress can lead to a zinc deficiency. I recommend supplementation of 30–60 milligrams daily with this mineral.

Botanicals. There are a number of herbal supplements I recommend. As I have already mentioned, my favorite is maca. Others that are particularly helpful for women under stress are quercetin, resveratrol, and grape seed extract. Another one I love is curcumin (derived from turmeric), which can reverse harmful effects of chronic stress. Medicinal mushrooms such as reishi are also beneficial.

Adrenal glandulars. These extracts are formulated with actual adrenal gland tissue usually derived from bovine (beef) sources. They help human adrenal glands repair themselves so they can heal and function normally again. An adrenal glandular can be a good source of adrenal support for mild to moderate cases of adrenal fatigue. Follow the manufacturer's recommendation for dosage.

Bioidentical adrenal support hormones. In addition to adrenal glandulars, another good option is to supplement with DHEA and pregnenolone. Both are normally secreted by the adrenals and may help to stimulate the adrenals to begin working normally again.

Before supplementing with oral DHEA, however, have your levels tested. If your DHEA-S (not DHEA) level is low (under 120 µg/dL), I recommend beginning treatment with 5 milligrams of DHEA per day and slowly working up to what feels like an optimal level to you (usually not above 15 milligrams) while doing the other adrenal-boosting activities. Your physician should be able to help you adjust your dosage accordingly.

For pregnenolone, I often use a progesterone topical cream that has 20 milligrams of progesterone and 10 milligrams of pregnenolone per pump dosage, applied in the evening at bedtime.

Note: It is best to work with a functional medicine doctor when you are struggling and get tested and your hormones and supplements customized for your personal needs. (To search for a functional doctor, see the Resources section.)

Practice a Daily Spiritual Assessment

For a long time I have done a kind of daily inventory of my spiritual health that is loosely based on the "Daily Examen" by St. Ignatius Loyola, a Spanish Basque priest and theologian. Now I've expanded my reflections and try to ask myself the following questions as a way to feel peace, check in with my stress levels and outlook, and hold myself accountable:

- Where did I see God/goodness or love today?
- Where could I have been more kind, patient, or loving today?
- What am I grateful for today?
- Where could I have laughed at myself more today? (That list is usually longer than I would like it to be!)
- How did I nourish myself today, physically, emotionally, and spiritually?
- Did I act based on love or on fear today?

Try this yourself. It is very powerful. Simply sit in a quiet place without interruptions, open yourself to the feeling of love, then ask yourself the questions above. Review your day with gratitude and look optimistically toward tomorrow; after all, it doesn't have any mistakes in it yet.

Consider EMDR and EFT

An American Psychological Association–approved therapy, eye movement desensitization and reprocessing (EMDR) works by engaging similar brain mechanisms as those that underpin rapid eye movement (REM) sleep. It is most often used to treat PTSD, in which symptoms of constant fear and panic follow a devastating event, but it has been so effective in many other areas of mental health.

During a typical session, you recall a troublesome memory (starting with a mild one, then working up to more traumatic memories). You then assign a number to the feeling of anxiety and apprehension associated with that memory, and identify any area in your body that may be holding tension or pain in association with that memory. Next, you'll hold that memory while watching a series of flashing lights or following a therapist's finger in front of your face from eye to eye, twelve to twenty-four times, re-creating the REM that occurs naturally in sleep. You're supportively guided through painful memories long enough to process and resolve them. EMDR causes you to remember the trauma, but in a calmer, more removed way. For instance, a rape victim may begin by feeling, *I'm no good. I feel ashamed and guilty.* At the end of treatment, she feels, *The shame is the rapist's, not mine. I'm a strong, resilient woman.*

At the end of each session, you're instructed to take a deep breath and then discuss your emotions or any other memory that crops up. You then move on to the next memory when you feel satisfied that the first no longer has a strong physical and/or emotional hold on you. EMDR works dramatically, though it is not clear why. It seems like the unprocessed memory is tucked away. Brain scans pre- and post-EMDR have shown increases in hippocampal volume in the brain. The hippocampus is a region of the brain associated with memory, emotions, and motivation. I've found EMDR to be very effective for myself and for many of my patients. They've been able to quickly heal old wounds and positively reset their physiology. It's like speed therapy!

Another helpful tool is Emotional Freedom Technique (EFT), which also helps heal psychological trauma. I've used EFT with myself and with my patients. The theory behind it is that blockages in the body's energy systems actually cause distress, and that tapping key points on your energy pathways can remove these blockages and the associated distress.

In a typical EFT session, you talk about your problem with a therapist or coach, followed by a description of the symptoms you experience when you think of that problem. Typically, your therapist asks you to rate the symptoms on a scale of 0 to 10, depending on the distress you feel. Then the therapist will have you tap on key acupressure points while focusing on specific emotional issues. As the therapy proceeds, you'll do more tapping as you think about the stress and rate your distress. In most cases, your number will have dropped.

Create a Resilient Heart

As an obstetrician, I have spent years listening to babies' heartbeats in utero and paying close attention to heart rate variability (HRV), the beat-to-beat fluctuations in heart rate. We listen and look for a high heart rate variability in order to reassure us that a baby is doing well. High HRV is a good sign of well-being and resilience. Low heart rate variability, on the other hand, is a sign of a stressed baby and stressed heart. At that point, we move quickly to get the baby delivered.

Through my own healing, I came to realize how important HRV is to adults too. When you are feeling calm and relaxed, HRV goes up, and you can more effortlessly manage stress. In healthy people, HRV is high. A high HRV determines your cardiovascular health, your fitness level, even your longevity. I have found consistently low HRV in clients under chronic stress and with PTSD.

Knowing this, we can do simple biofeedback training to improve HRV.

The HeartMath Institute (heartmath.org) has a website that offers great resources and an app called Inner Balance that requires a sensor. It takes you through various meditations and exercises with it. There are also now free or inexpensive apps for smartphones that use your camera and its flashlight tool. Just search "HRV" on your phone's app store.

Keep practicing and improve your HRV. Naturally, you'll want to do everything you can to raise it. Here are some other suggestions:

Try yoga. According to a study published in the *International Journal of Medical Engineering and Informatics* in 2010, HRV levels are higher in people who practice yoga than in nonpractitioners. Yoga is definitely a stress reliever. It is also excellent for flexibility and strength, and it is low-impact. It may also lower cortisol and bring you peace and centeredness.

I particularly like yoga because it bends and stretches you in all directions. If you're not fond of yoga for whatever reason, make sure you're wiggling, bending, shaking, and reaching out in all directions each day. Have fun while doing this—and sweat for its detox benefits.

Get grounded. "Grounding," also known as "earthing," elevates HRV. Grounding involves going barefoot outside, gardening, or swimming in the ocean. Other ways to ground include camping, hiking, or walking on the beach.

The Earth has a natural energy field. When you have physical contact with its surface, you absorb its natural healing energy. A study in *Journal of Environmental and Public Health* in 2012 demonstrated how grounding improves HRV by counteracting stress. It calms the autonomic nervous system, which regulates functions such as heart and respiration rates and digestion. An added benefit to grounding is that you will necessarily be outside to do it, which increases your exposure to sunlight and the all-important vitamin D that's created by the body when skin is exposed to sunlight.

Limit exposure to electromagnetic fields (EMFs). Overexposure to the electro-pollution of radio frequencies (which typically come from cell towers, cordless telephones, and cellphones) can reduce HRV, says a 2009 study in the *International Archives of Occupational and Environmental Health*. Consider ways to reduce your exposure: Limit the number and duration of cellphone calls. Turn off your router at night. And unplug electrical equipment when not in use. Stand back from your microwave while cooking. Try not to live near cell towers and high-tension power lines. Put your phone in airplane mode unless you are expecting a call.

Relax with music. Soothing music helps deepen your breathing, which elevates HRV, say researchers writing in *Alternative Therapies in Health and Medicine* in 2015. Slow-tempo classical music is best. But select music that you like and truly relaxes you. If you don't care for Beethoven, for example, it likely won't have a positive effect on your HRV. We play lullaby instrumental music at bedtime more for me than my daughter.

Think positively. Negative thinking isn't just bad for your mood, it's also bad for your brain and your hormone balance. Chronic anger, hate, and resentment produce stress, causing your adrenals to release too much cortisol. Over time, high levels of cortisol shrink the hippocampus (the brain area associated with memory and emotions) and can cause more negative thinking.

I understand that you can't always remove stressors from your life. But maybe you can change your perceptions and responses to some of them. As Dale Carnegie once said, "Everybody in the world is seeking happiness, and there is one sure way to find it. That is by controlling your thoughts. Happiness doesn't depend on outward conditions. It depends on inward conditions."

That quote reminds me of something a professor in medical school said to me: "You are the only one who can upset yourself."

I had protested, "No, my boyfriend can really piss me off!"

To which he had responded, "No, *you choose how to respond*. You are in control of your emotions."

I have kept that as a strong reminder—which is why I recommend reframing your negative thoughts whenever they bubble up. Ask yourself, "Is there another way of seeing this thought or situation? How would my best friend look at this thought? Is there a silver lining?" This helps you transform negative thoughts into positive ones.

One of my favorite Bible verses is Philippians 4:8: "Whatever is true, whatever is noble, whatever is right, whatever is pure, whatever is lovely, whatever is admirable—if anything is excellent or praiseworthy—think about such things." That passage is the essence of positive thinking.

Pause. Breathe. Smile. Connect. I put myself through college by working multiple jobs. I went to medical school and worked one hundred hours per week during my residency. Then I became a busy obstetrician, wife, and mother. I couldn't have done all that without being a consummate multitasker! But after years of living life as an overstressed multitasker, I finally started living the following mantra: *Pause. Breathe. Smile. Connect.* When you breathe deeply, your vagus nerve—it starts at the back of your head and runs all the way through your body—tells your brain to get into relaxation mode. When you smile, there's a measurable reduction in your blood pressure. Smiling releases endorphins (natural painkillers) and the feel-good hormone serotonin. Smiling lifts your face and makes you look years younger. Smiling makes us feel good and look good. It is a natural uplifting drug. Also, if we have to have wrinkles, I'd rather have smile and laugh lines than frowny lines.

Then there is connection. To me this means not answering a phone call or text while cooking dinner or spending time with my family. A car ride with my kids is phone-free time.

It would be unreasonable to completely forgo our electronic devices to spend endless time with our families, or stop multitasking altogether. All I'm suggesting is a little moderation. We don't have to be enslaved to modern life. We get to choose. Choose simplicity.

I choose by designating certain times of the day when I give loved ones and friends my full attention. For example, I spend uninterrupted time with my ten-year-old daughter before she goes to sleep. I leave my phone outside the room and in airplane mode. This is a very sacred time for us, and I cherish it. Our loved ones need to know we are listening to them and that they have our attention too. This fuels our spirit as well.

These one-on-one connections actually increase our "love and bonding" hormone oxytocin. It is released when we connect with other people. We'll get more into detail about oxytocin in Chapter 11, but for now understand this: When cortisol goes up, oxytocin goes down. This combination makes menopause a more difficult transition than it has to be. So part of the solution is to boost oxytocin and normalize cortisol through love, bonding, gratitude, a positive outlook, close family, and social connections. When we have those, we are more resilient and our passage through menopause is easier.

This is your time to smile and laugh more, connect with loved ones, take the time to eat healthy meals, take long luxurious baths, and discover new things. Nurture a positive outlook and be grateful for day-to-day blessings. When you adopt these ways of thinking, being, and living, you can control the impact of hormonal shifts on your life and move forward to the next great phase of your beautiful life while enjoying all the present moments.

Chapter 9

Vaginal Health: Get Your Sexy Back

Your vagina is essential for life. I've made this announcement at international medical conferences with more than four hundred male physicians in attendance. Their reaction: some laughs and many eye rolls!

Regardless, it is true. We wouldn't be here if women didn't have vaginas. Our children's lives begin there. Sexual pleasure and bonding happen there. The vagina is also a window to our overall health, revealing pH, hormone imbalances, gut problems, and much more. The vagina, and indeed the whole vulvar area, is a key aspect of our femininity and should be embraced as such—not ignored or neglected.

After your hormones begin changing, your health "down there" starts changing. Even though you might be embarrassed to talk to your gynecologist about this (don't be—we've seen and heard it all), you can't afford to ignore the changes.

Maybe you can relate to Julie, a fifty-seven-year-old teacher. She was really struggling at this time of her life. She felt her second marriage was about to fall apart. She had zero sex drive. She told me, "And what's worse, I leak urine when I try to exercise." She also leaked urine when she coughed or sneezed, and the urgency was restricting her love of "just doing stuff."

After further questioning, I learned that she also suffered with vaginal dryness and irritation after sex, "the few times we've had it in the past year," and a total lack of energy. As she said, "My get-up-and-go got up and left!"

Like Julie, you too may be going through age- and hormone-related changes that are interfering with sexual functioning, leading to vaginal dryness, libido problems, and bladder struggles. Good news: The right nutrients, a healthy lifestyle, and targeted natural remedies can prevent or relieve the most common ailments associated with vaginal changes. That's why we've got to talk about how to handle the vaginal issues you're facing, and learn how to stay healthy—and sexy—for years to come.

Vaginal Atrophy: Its Life-Altering Symptoms

Declining hormone levels lead to vaginal atrophy, which is very common during and after menopause but also experienced in our thirties and forties as well. This happens when vaginal tissue gets thinner, less lubricated, and less elastic. Muscle loss also occurs. Women can't readily see tissue changes that are otherwise easily visible to a physician. But if you've noticed thin lines on your face and around your lips, it is happening on your lower lips (labia) too.

You are not alone. With aging, menopause, and hormonal changes, approximately 75 percent of postmenopausal women suffer from vaginal atrophy. It causes:

- Painful intercourse due to decreased lubrication or excessive vaginal dryness
- A higher rate of vaginal and bladder infections (due to imbalances and decline of normal vaginal bacteria and increased pH)
- Leaking urine
- Decreased desire, arousal, and orgasm

Women tend to mistake their symptoms for common irritations, allergies, or infections. More often, the changes are so gradual that the symptoms go unnoticed for years until there is pain, discharge, or incontinence. Unlike hot flashes, which usually end even without treatment, vaginal atrophy symptoms usually increase in severity over time.

Consider this: The current life expectancy for American women is more than eighty years (based on 2010 census data) and continues to increase. Given that menopause starts, on average, at around fifty-one, women may live almost 40 percent of their entire lives in this discomfort and decreased quality of life. Forty percent of our lives living with this misery? Unacceptable!

Yet, it's happening. An analysis of responses from my Eve Quiz (see page 23) shows that:

- 70 percent of women said they had issues with arousal
- 64 percent of women had troublesome vaginal or vulvar dryness
- About 62 percent of women noted some discomfort during or after sex
- Just under 70 percent of women said they had experienced urinary leakage when coughing, sneezing, and the like

Painful numbers, right? We can improve so much of this. We just need to understand what is happening to our bodies.

Down-There Dryness

With menopause and natural aging, your vagina slows down production of its normal, healthy secretions. You're dry "down there," and often it's difficult or painful to have intercourse. But once you take action to resolve dryness, you'll feel sexually reborn and your libido will return.

Steps to Solve It

1. Minimize toxic exposures to your delicate lady parts. One of the most common causes of vaginal and vulvar irritations is related to the wide variety of personal care products we may use such as bubble baths, perfumed soaps, fragrances, feminine wash, and personal lubricants. These can all be very irritating. They may cause allergic reactions and may even expose you to nasty

hormone-disrupting chemicals, so please read labels and be aware of ingredients such as parabens. Tampons, liners, and pads can also be laden with hormone-disrupting chemicals and GMOs. They can also cause tissue trauma and irritation.

2. Include essential fats and probiotics in your diet. By following the Keto-Green Diet and lifestyle, you'll automatically be feeding your body these vital nutrients. This diet includes healthy fatty foods such as salmon (wild-caught), oysters, eggs from free-range chickens, avocados, organic butter from free-range cows, and olive oil—all of which help your body naturally create hormones. Eat fermented foods, such as sauerkraut, and cultured foods, such as Greek yogurt (if you eat dairy), which are rich in probiotics, and supplement with a good probiotic. Probiotics support healthy bacteria in your vagina. (See the Resources section for probiotic recommendations.)

3. Use *natural* lubricants and vaginal moisturizing creams. Non-hormonal vaginal lubricants and moisturizers help reduce dryness. Lubricants are applied just before sex; moisturizers are applied more regularly, for longer-term relief. Both are helpful, but they do not "cure" vaginal dryness and other symptoms of atrophy. Even so, consider natural options like Good Clean Love and Yes products. Both are paraben-free with clean ingredients and come in both water-based and oil-based options.

4. Try herbal and natural therapies. Over-the-counter herbal remedies typically contain black cohosh, soy isoflavones, magnolia bark, maca (my favorite), and other herbal ingredients. Products formulated with isoflavones have been heavily marketed to address vaginal dryness symptoms. In 2003, one study showed that soy-rich diets increase the maturation indices of vaginal cells (a measure of the health of the vagina) and deemed such diets an effective preventive intervention against vaginal atrophy.

Some of the natural supplements on the market are Estroven, which contains black cohosh, soy isoflavones, magnolia bark, and other herbs, and Remifemin, an herbal supplement containing a standardized extract of black cohosh root. These, however, may not be appropriate for women dealing with breast cancer, since isoflavones are associated with an increase in excess estrogen. Soy products may also contain soy that has been genetically modified, so I always caution choosing dietary non-GMO options such as miso, tempeh, and natto.

There are also natural lubricant solutions, including organic coconut oil, ayurvedic ghee (ghee infused with certain herbs), or an organic lubricant. These do not contain the additional chemicals but offer satisfactory moisturizing benefits.

MAKE YOUR OWN VAGINAL LUBRICANT

Ingredients

¼ cup fractionated organic coconut oil (a liquid coconut oil that has had the longer-chain fatty acids removed; check the label)

¼ cup aloe gel

1–4 drops essential oil*

Directions

Combine all ingredients in a glass jar. Shake well.

Keep by your bedside, and use as much as desired prior to and during intimacy or with intimate massage.

---

* A few essential oils that I like to mix in with my DIY lubricant, and ones shown to soothe vaginal tissues, include clary sage, Roman chamomile (*Anthemis nobilis*) or Cape chamomile (*Eriocephalus punctulatus*), rose, lavender, frankincense, and sandalwood. A word of caution: never apply essential oils directly on the vaginal or vulvar skin. Always use a carrier oil or the recipe above, and before using in the vaginal area, test on your inner arm skin first for signs of irritation.

---

5. Use topical DHEA. While most research and available treatments for vaginal dryness have focused on estrogen, DHEA has

also been found to play an important role in addressing the issue (and many other vaginal atrophy symptoms). As estrogen levels naturally decrease with age, it is DHEA that continues to be a remaining primary source of estrogens and androgens in your body. But there is a progressive decrease in serum DHEA starting in your midtwenties and an average 60 percent loss by menopause.

It's important to note that while oral DHEA and oral estrogen are used for a variety of other health benefits, neither has been shown to address vaginal dryness or other vaginal atrophy symptoms satisfactorily.

Topical DHEA is a different story. The research surrounding vaginally applied prescription forms of DHEA has shown that it:

- Reduces vaginal dryness and irritation and improves vaginal pH
- Strengthens vaginal musculature
- Increases bone mineral density
- Decreases pain during intercourse
- Increases arousal and libido, as well as sexual satisfaction

I have routinely seen positive results in my medical practice since 1999 as well: improvements to sexual health and vaginal dryness, a reduction in irritation and pain during intercourse, and regular improvements in libido and sexual satisfaction. Some patients also reported decreased incontinence symptoms. Many patients who originally came to see me for possible surgery due to pelvic prolapse and incontinence were able to avoid surgery altogether once I prescribed vaginal DHEA and testosterone to them.

A good example is Venessa, who was sixty-two when she came to my office complaining of vaginal pain and urgency incontinence symptoms. She had had a hysterectomy when she was thirty due to endometriosis. At fifty-five she had undergone vaginal surgery for prolapse and pelvic floor relaxation, called a cystocoele and rectocoele repair. This is done by suturing in the vaginal walls.

Not only did Venessa have what she called a "stabbing" vaginal pain, but she just didn't feel well. She had lost her intimacy with her husband, was tired, and couldn't lose weight. She was also on multiple medications, including two cholesterol-lowering drugs, an antacid, the anti-inflammatories tramadol and aspirin, and vaginal estrogen twice per week—all without relief.

The exam I did and the labs I ordered noted significant vaginal and clitoral shrinkage and a suture that had eroded through the vaginal lining. All of these conditions were the source of her pain, along with dryness and scarring. Her abdomen was quite bloated, and her skin was very dry.

My passion and concern for women's health care and my own life lessons taught me to take a functional, head-to-toe approach with clients like Venessa. So my assessment and recommendations for her were:

- Get Keto-Green, starting with a low-carb, alkalinizing, gluten-free, grain-free diet to stop inflammation and gastrointestinal issues.
- Consume more detoxifying veggies (such as estrogen-detoxifying cruciferous vegetables) and eliminate processed foods.
- Take a thyroid supplement (Nature-Throid ½ grain), along with selenium, iodine, and zinc. Eat two Brazil nuts nightly (which would provide approximately 200 micrograms of selenium); oysters, because they are rich in zinc and tyrosine; and sushi or seaweed for natural iodine. (Venessa's thyroid function was not at its peak, based on her hormonal panel—and these supplements and foods would help her.)
- Wean off antacids. I added probiotics and digestive enzymes to her daily regimen.
- I asked her to focus on chewing her food until it dissolved in her mouth (a first step in supporting digestion) and to not drink more than 4 ounces of fluid with meals to allow her digestive enzymes to work.

- I recommended that Venessa take vaginal hormones for a month prior to surgery for her vaginal erosion, suture perforation, dryness, and pain.
- Do Kegel exercises for her pelvic floor (see the information on page 176).
- Seek counseling for stress and concern for her marital relationship.

Prior to Venessa's one-month follow-up appointment, something funny and a little embarrassing happened. I ran into Venessa and her husband in an airport. She introduced me to her husband, saying, "Honey, this is Dr. Anna Cabeca. Thanks to her, I've had the best orgasms and am feeling frisky again! And no more migraines!" She was truly amazed how much better she felt.

Venessa followed up with me the next week, so I could reexamine her and do her pre-op for surgery. I was hopeful there would be healthier tissue so I could do a good surgical repair. Well, on exam, her vaginal lining had completely healed. The suture was no longer visible or tender! Her vagina looked twenty years younger! There was no need to do surgery. You can imagine how thrilled she was!

NECESSITY IS THE MOTHER OF INVENTION

Women suffer needlessly and silently with vulvar and vaginal issues that really can decrease quality and enjoyment of life. Vulvar and vaginal dryness leads often to incontinence too. It became my mission to create a better solution—a safe, easy nonprescription treatment that addressed quality of life and health issues associated with menopause and aging of our lady parts.

After three intense years of research and testing, I developed a topical anti-aging vulvar cream called Julva, formulated with DHEA and other quality natural ingredients shown to be beneficial to the skin and its underlying tissues. Those key ingredients include alpine rose stem cells, emu oil, vitamin E, coconut oil, and shea butter. This combination works better than anything else I have ever tried or prescribed.

Alpine rose stem cells are particularly interesting and helpful. They contain unique compounds that help the plant survive in extremely challenging environments. The stem cells have been shown to increase skin cell moisture, protect against age-related oxidative stress, and confer antiviral effects. They are also loaded with antioxidant compounds.

You can find out more about Julva at dranna.com/resources, and decide for yourself if you would like to try it. If you do, my research shows that a small (pea-size) amount daily of Julva topically applied to the vulva achieves excellent improvements.

"Ouch, Darling": Painful Intercourse

You might feel pain during sex, both on the inside of your vagina and externally on the labia, clitoris, and vaginal opening—and it can happen at any age. There can be other causes besides menopause. For instance, antihistamines can cause vaginal dryness and pain, so if you're taking them, ask your doctor about other options. Other conditions such as fibroids and endometriosis can also cause pain during sex, so see your doctor to identify any underlying concerns. Consider it a great reason to get a harmless pelvic ultrasound to assess your uterus and ovaries too. So see your gynecologist. It's always important to get to the root cause.

The same strategies I discussed in the preceding section help address painful intercourse as well, since it is caused by vaginal dryness. In addition, watch your exposure to toxins, go Keto-Green, lubricate and moisturize your vagina, and use topical DHEA regularly. In addition, here are some other steps you can take for painful intercourse.

1. Obviously, the first step is to get clear on what is causing the pelvic discomfort or pain. Get a gynecologic exam, pelvic sono-

gram, and wet prep (a microscopic evaluation of the vaginal milieu) or Ubiome vaginal microbiota test.

2. If the dryness is from age-related hormone decline, talk to your gynecologist about vaginal androgens. Please understand that many physicians may not yet be comfortable with prescribing vaginal androgens for women or prescribing customized compounded bioidentical hormones, but it really is my recommendation to find a doctor who has experience and confidence in doing so.

In November 2016, the FDA approved a DHEA vaginal suppository called Intrarosa (prasterone), which has undergone extensive research and has a great safety profile. If that is not an option for you, local low-dose estrogen helps many women with vaginal atrophy, and thus eases painful intercourse. It comes in some bioidentical prescription creams (such as Estrace), a small tablet inserted in the vagina (Vagifem), and a flexible vaginal ring that's worn continuously (Estring). Vaginal application releases a tiny amount of estrogen into the bloodstream. It carries less risk of side effects than systemic (oral) hormone therapy.

Estrogen products help improve the thickness and elasticity of the vaginal mucosal lining but do not appear to affect the deeper tissue or supporting muscles. Rather than just temporarily adding moisture (like the lubricants of the previous section), they actually work to reverse the thinning and dryness of vaginal tissue; these benefits may alleviate painful sexual intercourse.

Additionally, estrogen and androgens can help with vaginal pH by adding some moisture back, which can help support the normal vaginal flora and bacteria, but the effect appears to be small.

It is my long-term preference—based on clinical and scientific experience and research—that hormone replacement should only be bioidentical and in the lowest effective dose initially to achieve best results. This is true for replacement of all hormones, including progesterone, estrogen, testosterone, and

DHEA. Working with compounding pharmacies and natural ingredients to customize individual treatments has always been my preference.

Incontinence: Laugh, Cough, Pee . . . Repeat

Starting as early as our twenties and increasing over time, many of us will suffer from urinary incontinence—the involuntary loss of bladder control. In results from my Eve Questionnaire, nearly 70 percent of women said they had experienced urinary leakage when coughing, sneezing, and the like. Urinary incontinence not only causes us to lose our feminine confidence and daily comfort but also negatively impacts our sexual relationships.

There are four main types of urinary incontinence I'd like to discuss here:

Overactive bladder. Also called urgency incontinence and known medically as detrusor instability, this is a problem with the muscles and nerves in the bladder. A common sign that you might have an overactive bladder is that you typically have the urge to run to the bathroom, and may even urinate a little before you get there. Older women tend to experience this quite frequently but it occurs in youth as well.

Nocturia. When you have to use the bathroom at night, once, twice, even three times, you may have nocturia. I had one client who used to get up six times every night to use the bathroom. That was simply untenable if for no other reason than she was never getting a good and full night's rest. Because it also affects older women, nocturia is risky since it involves getting up at night, when most falls and hip fractures occur.

Post-void dribbling. After you feel like you've emptied your bladder, you get up from the toilet and leak a bit. This is post-void dribbling, which occurs when your bladder is not emptying completely or from a weakness in the urethra, which is where you urinate from.

Stress urinary incontinence. This kind of leakage occurs when you put any kind of stress on your bladder, such as coughing, sneezing, laughing, or even exercising.

Painful urination. This is not a form of urinary incontinence, but it is important to discuss because it occurs in many women who are in hormonal decline. If it burns or stings when you urinate, get a urine analysis because you may have a bladder infection or something else that needs to be fixed.

Lifestyle has a lot to do with our risk factors for incontinence as well:

Diet. Several beverages can worsen incontinence, such as caffeine, carbonated drinks, and alcohol. Spicy foods do too, because they stimulate or irritate the bladder. So avoiding these foods can make a big difference.

Childbirth. Experts disagree how much this directly impacts the development of incontinence. (Based on my clinical practice, however, I'd say pregnancy and natural childbirth do create wear and tear, especially the more pregnancies you have, whether delivered vaginally or by cesarean section.)

Hormonal decline. As we get older, our hormones decline, and with that we lose collagen, a protein that provides structure for our tissues. We also lose muscle strength around the bladder, further contributing to incontinence.

Obesity. Being very overweight can boost your risk for developing incontinence issues because of the associated increased intra-abdominal pressure and inflammation.

Drugs. Certain medications such as diuretics can cause incontinence symptoms by promoting the output of urine and relaxing bladder musculature.

Regardless of what specific kind of leakage or incontinence you have, if it keeps you from doing the things you love to do or getting the rest you need, it's a real problem.

It's very important that we prevent urinary problems for the long haul. In older people with serious health issues, urinary incontinence can add to the reasons that make it difficult for caregivers to continue to care for them at home. I don't plan to give my kids any additional reason to tuck me away somewhere when I'm older! And we don't want to have to wear pads or panty liners with our sexy undies, do we?

There are proven solutions to this problem—and they don't involve drugs or surgery.

1. Watch what you eat. Omit foods that stimulate the bladder: caffeine, sugar, processed foods, artificial sweeteners, and preservatives in food. Foods that cause allergies and sensitivities can be offenders too: gluten, dairy, eggs, soy, tree nuts, and certain other foods such as peanuts. If problems continue after eliminating these foods, see your doctor for additional food sensitivity testing. And choose healthy whole Keto-Green foods, including alkaline foods and healthy fats such as those found in avocados, salmon, and oysters.

2. Maintain a healthy weight. Research demonstrates that weight loss is a first-line treatment for incontinence. In a randomized study of forty-seven overweight or moderately obese women with urinary incontinence, participants decreased their incontinence episodes by 53 percent following a three-month weight loss program. If you get on the Keto-Green program, you can maintain the healthiest weight for you—and reduce the possibility of urinary incontinence.

3. Supplement your diet. If you have recurrent urinary tract infections, for example, take vitamin C, 4,000 milligrams daily. Supplementation can greatly reduce your risk of further infections or irritations to your bladder. However, in some women, vitamin C can actually make urinary problems worse, so you have to listen to your body and figure out what works best for you. Sometimes just a different brand or buffered vitamin C is better tolerated.

   Other supplements to make sure you're taking include magnesium and probiotics. I believe that a good probiotic is a great line of defense against digestive issues and inflammation in the body (including inflammation relating to our sexual health). If you have been diagnosed with small intestine bacterial overgrowth (SIBO), do not take probiotics, because you must get rid of the overgrowth first.

4. Consider bioidentical hormone therapy. I've observed this to be very effective in relieving urinary incontinence. Talk to your doctor about topical or intravaginal bioidentical hormones to help improve your symptoms.

5. Ask your doctor for a prescription for compounded vulvar vaginal DHEA and/or testosterone. Or use Julva—it contains restorative ingredients and plant stem cells to help repair the delicate tissue and mucous membranes around the urethra, vagina, and rectum.

6. Keep a "bladder journal." When are you having the problem? Is your issue at night? Do you experience it while you are doing certain things like exercising? Have you just had something in particular to eat or drink? (Eliminating diuretic beverages such as coffee and tea, as well as bladder irritants such as citrus juice and sugars, might be of help.) Do you feel like you absolutely have to pee, but then you don't once you have the chance? All of this info will be handy for you to discuss with your doctor.

7. Try bladder retraining. Your doctor may suggest you attempt to work at retraining your bladder to address issues with urge incontinence. Timed voiding and holding the urine for a few minutes after you feel the urge and then slowly increasing the intervals over a period of time may be of help.

8. Perform pelvic floor exercises. When you think of exercise, you probably think about working the muscles of your back, legs, and arms. But your pelvic floor muscles are super-important too, because they're involved in bladder and bowel control, as well as sexual function (including arousal and orgasm). Kegel or pelvic floor exercises strengthen the pubococcygeus muscles of the pelvic floor by alternately contracting and relaxing them.

   Although the exercises are highly effective to help prevent or treat urinary incontinence, Kegel exercises can also help prevent prolapse, a condition in which the pelvic organs slip from their normal position. If you already have prolapse, performing Kegels won't cure the condition; however, doing them regularly stops its progression.

How to Perform Kegel Exercises

Think of your pelvic floor muscles—the muscles you squeeze when you're trying to stop the flow of pee while urinating—as a "hammock," holding everything up. They need to be strong or you're likely to experience incontinence as well as pelvic prolapse—so exercise them!

But first, determine how strong your pelvic muscles are right now. Do a quick self-test by trying to stop your urine midstream while peeing, and hold for a count of 10. If you can't stop your urine stream, your pelvic floor muscles are not as strong as they should be. Don't repeat this test too often, however. It can work against your muscle control. Just do it to initially test yourself. Then repeat it a week after implementing Kegels. Self-test infrequently after that.

Here's how to do the perfect Kegels:

1. Lie down on your side, so that you're not putting pressure on your pelvic floor.
2. Pinpoint your perineal muscles—the general region between your vagina and anus.
3. Contract the muscles by squeezing (contracting) them and holding for a count of 3 on an exhale. Breathe normally, then relax for ten seconds and repeat. Eventually work up to holding for a count of 6 or 8.
4. Establish a routine where you do 10 to 20 Kegels daily three times per week. The total time you spend doing them is a mere five minutes a day.
5. Try using jade eggs or Kegel balls to strengthen your vaginal muscles.

There are other exercises helpful for pelvic health:

- Walking is a great daily exercise. Just maintain good posture while you're walking.
- Do hip circles. Stand and keep your shoulders still while rotating just your hips (kind of like a hula dancer). Imagine you are drawing a circle on the floor with your hips. Draw a small circle and then a larger one. This activates the lower area of your core, which strengthens all of the muscles in that area.
- Incorporate stretching into your weekly routine. Yoga is a great therapy to keep your hips, pelvic floor, and core strong and healthy.

I have a video about pelvic floor exercises on my website that's very informative and instructive. Check out dranna.com/resources.

WHAT ABOUT SURGERY?

A number of surgeries are available to treat vaginal atrophy and incontinence. Should you go that route? My overriding advice is to try natural treatments first, including supplements, diet, pelvic exercises, Julva, and bioidentical hormones. Surgery should be considered as a last resort, when everything else has failed. I wrote an ebook devoted to this topic: *All Things V.* You can download it from my website.

Don't Forget a Vaginal Self-Exam

Just as it's important to do regular breast self-exams to check for lumps or other changes, it is also important to do vaginal self-exams for early detection of issues. If you find a problem, you can start treatment sooner, and you'll more likely have a better outcome.

A self-exam isn't as in-depth as a pelvic exam performed by your gynecologist. But it may help you find signs of sexually transmitted disease or changes to your vulva (the outer part of your genitals) that could indicate other health problems.

To do the exam, get a handheld mirror, a flashlight or other small light, pillows, and a towel.

Take your clothes off from your waist down. Sit on your bed or on a towel on the floor. Sit with your back propped up by pillows, in a butterfly position (feet pulled toward your butt and legs spread). Then examine the parts of your vulva: the clitoris and the outer and inner labia. Take note of anything unusual.

Gently spread the labia apart and angle the mirror and light so you can see into your vagina. The walls should be pinkish in color, elastic, and non-tender. If during your vaginal self-exam you see any genital warts, sores, bumps, or pale or unusual discoloration, make an appointment to see your doctor.

You have so many natural options to restore your vaginal health and reverse atrophy. I've treated many women who initially thought they needed surgery for a gynecological problem, only to find that once I put them on natural therapies or hormones for a few weeks (to ensure their vaginal tissue was optimal for surgery) that they no longer needed the surgery! I encourage you to speak to your doctor if you are experiencing incontinence or other sexual health issues. But remember there are natural-care actions you can take first to improve your health "down there."

Chapter 10

Rejuvenate Your Routine:
Movement and Sleep

Once upon a time, menopause was seen as the end of our vital years. But as I have pointed out, the end of our periods opens up a door (just as the start of them did), and these changes can be the beginning of a vibrant new life—an exciting transition. And what you do during this time can shape your physical and emotional life for years to come. If in reasonably good health, women who make smart choices in menopause are more likely to live longer, healthier lives. Remember, life is nowhere near over—in fact, it can be better than ever. It's our choice to walk through this door and enthusiastically reclaim our lives.

As you have learned, the smartest choice of all is staying Keto-Green because of the way it affects the balance of insulin, cortisol, and oxytocin. Other smart choices that impact this balance are exercise and sleep.

Fix Hormones with Exercise

Exercise is an excellent hormone fix. A number of studies demonstrate that many of the changes—both physical and mental—that we associate with aging and menopause are partly the result of inactivity. And many of the women I have worked with over the years—women who began exercising during menopause—tell me that it changed their lives.

Hormonally, oxytocin increases when you exercise. Excess cortisol is dissipated. With exercise helping the body to consume cortisol and other stress hormones such as epinephrine and norepinephrine, the result is a decrease in blood pressure, heart rate, and anxiety. Exercise makes your muscles more receptive to insulin, so you're less likely to become insulin resistant. Endorphins—the feel-good hormones—are released during exercise and have been shown to have an effect in regulating blood pressure and body temperature. They may also have a role in controlling your appetite too.

More broadly speaking, there are other irrefutable benefits of exercise during menopause:

- Your heart will be stronger.
- Your bone density will be greater.
- You will have more energy and stamina.
- You will naturally detox your system.
- Your mood will lift and you will get a positive feeling about your body and your life.
- You will reduce the frequency and intensity of hot flashes.
- You will fight creeping fat gain, especially around your middle.
- You may prevent dementia.

The Best Exercise?

Everyone always wants to know, what kind of exercise is best? My answer: Whatever you love and will stick to! Have you tried belly dancing, Zumba, or hooping? These are fabulous exercises that get you moving your hips, which will keep you flexible and more mobile throughout your life—and they are very oxytocin-boosting!

Exercise has powerful benefits for all ages, and particularly if you are over fifty. Any type of exercise is better than none at all, so no matter what your state of fitness right now, do what you can. You can start gradually, adding a fifteen-minute walk to your daily routine, taking the stairs instead of the elevator, or starting the day with some calisthenics.

Tiny changes count. I've had many clients who began with a few extra steps and now run marathons. So it's important to persevere and not give up.

Personally, I love to do yoga, walk, weight-train, swim, play tennis, and box—and I do one of these practically every day. Because I exercise regularly, I feel better and I have more energy. Sometimes during the week I get busy and can't find the time. But when that happens, I miss it. I really do!

The research is clear—nothing turns back the clock and improves life and life expectancy like exercise.

Yoga, Hormones, and Menopause

I discussed yoga earlier as a way to relieve stress, but there is so much more to this ancient practice. The word "yoga" actually refers to a union of body, mind, and spirit, an alignment of the physical and nonphysical parts of yourself. It's not an overstatement: If you practice yoga, you will not only find your health and well-being improve, but every area of your life will benefit.

The research bears this out. One study published in 2016 in *Complementary Therapies in Medicine* involved eighty-eight postmenopausal women who were randomly assigned to one of three groups: control (no intervention), exercise, and yoga. They all filled out questionnaires about their menopausal symptoms, and the researchers did lab work to check levels of cortisol, follicle-stimulating hormone (FSH), luteinizing hormone (LH), progesterone, and estrogen.

After twelve weeks, the women who practiced yoga showed dramatically lower scores for menopausal symptoms, stress levels, and depression, as well as significantly higher scores in quality of life, when compared to the control and exercise groups. The control group presented a significant increase in cortisol levels. The yoga and exercise groups showed decreased levels of FSH and LH when compared to the control group. The researchers concluded that yoga would be a great complementary therapy for women undergoing hormonal changes with age. Yoga is a hormone fixer, for sure.

A 2016 study, published in *Topics in Geriatric Rehabilitation*, found that 80 percent of older participants, most of whom had osteoporosis or its precursor, osteopenia (low bone density), who practiced twelve yoga poses (often modified) a day showed improved bone density in their spine and femurs.* Each pose was held for thirty seconds. The daily regimen, once learned, took only twelve minutes to complete. These findings applied to younger women with healthy skeletons too.

I can see why. Yoga plays a vital role in preventing fractures by building stability, flexibility, and agility. This means you're less likely to fall and break something—and if you do start to fall, your agility may help you catch yourself.

Not only can yoga help to fight disease, but in many cases it can halt chronic illnesses such as arthritis, asthma, and many other conditions. Yoga activates the parasympathetic nervous system, which initiates the more tranquil functions of the body.

Yoga is definitely a legitimate, natural treatment for menopause symptoms. Yoga classes are available at practically all gyms, fitness centers, and community centers, so you should be able to easily enroll in a class that meets your needs and level of experience. No matter how time-crunched you are, you can create time for yoga. In fact, yoga will create more time for you.

Punch Your Way to Fitness

The idea of socking a punching bag after a stressful day at work sounded appealing to me—so I signed on with a trainer at my gym to put me through a thirty-minute boxing routine a couple of times a week. It's a great workout, because you use your entire body—shoulders, arms, abs, butt, and legs—to throw a punch. I started in 2007, and it is my preferred exercise. Plus, if you love wearing off-the-shoulder blouses, nothing else gives you great shoulders the way boxing does!

It doesn't take a long time to pick up the moves either. In my first session, I learned the proper position my body should be in before I even

---

* Doctors used to believe that women's ability to build new bone basically ended at menopause when their levels of bone-protective estrogen and progesterone plummeted. But new research shows that yoga is surprisingly protective when it comes to staving off fractures and helping to prevent osteoporosis, which will cause approximately half of women age 50 and older to break a bone.

tried to box. Then, with my feet placed correctly and my fists (in boxing gloves) clenched and slightly tilted inward in front of my face, I learned about straight punches, undercuts, and hooks.

Next, my trainer put on a pair of pads and encouraged me to punch them with my left fist, then my right. There was a lot to think about. While throwing a punch with my right fist, and getting the correct position with it, I had to remember to keep my face protected with my left hand.

Moving on, I faced my first punching bag. What an arm and shoulder workout! I was sore for days.

Then I did crunches in which I had to alternately punch my trainer's pads on the sit-up part of the move. We continued like that for thirty minutes in a circuit-type session. It was intense. Well, I was hardly Muhammad Ali, but with my trainer's watchful eye and encouragement I was feeling a lot more confident. I love it.

The benefits are astonishing—especially if you want to burn belly fat. Australian researchers compared the outcome of a high-intensity boxing routine performed four times a week to walking on a treadmill. The boxers trimmed their waistlines, plus lowered their blood pressure and felt more energized. The treadmill exercisers did not improve in any of these areas. In fact, they ran low on energy! This study was published in 2015 in the journal *BMC Sports Science, Medicine and Rehabilitation*.

Plus, punching stuff is like therapy. I call it my meditation because I am focused on placing my punches and can't really be distracted by anything else going on in my head. Also, though anger release isn't the reason I box, I have to admit that when I *kapow* the bag, stress-reducing hormones are dissipated throughout my body, and as a result, I feel calm and relieved.

These days it is relatively easy to learn how to box your way to fitness. Boxing circuit-training gyms that cater to regular exercisers are popping up all over the place. Plus, most gyms and fitness centers have boxing equipment such as punching bags. As I did, have a trainer take you through the fundamentals to get comfortable with correct form so you won't hurt yourself and will have fun.

Strong-Arm Hormones and Menopause

Strength training is essential for skeletal health, weight control, and overall well-being of women after menopause. Findings from the Study of Women's Health Across the Nation (SWAN), a study of ten thousand women as they go through menopause, showed that 20 to 30 percent of forty- to fifty-five-year-olds had difficulty performing simple physical tasks such as climbing a flight of stairs or carrying grocery bags around the block. Even putting clothes on over your head or clasping your bra strap can become difficult. If women are that weak then, what will happen to them at eighty?

Fortunately, various studies show that engaging in just two strength-training workouts a week increases strength in women over fifty quite significantly.

Lift weights, use strength-training machines, or do bodyweight functional exercises at least two days a week. Do one set each of ten to twelve moves that strengthen your major muscle groups—arms, shoulders, chest, back, abdominals, hips, and legs. If you're beginning, choose a lighter weight you can lift at least 15 to 20 times. Once this gets comfortable, and you are over the soreness, increase the weights to where you can do a maximum of only 10 to 12 reps.

The bottom line: Get active, find something you love, and do it regularly!

Sleep Your Way to a Hormone Fix

An essential lifestyle fix I recommend is to get a good night's sleep. I know this may seem easier said than done; I've had the toughest time with this lifestyle habit myself. Like most medical students, interns, residents, and doctors, I worked many hours and pulled many all-nighters. We are among the most sleep-deprived segment of the population, maybe even worse than new parents. The truth is that while I love to stay in bed, I was only getting three to five hours of sleep a night, and my PTSD aggravated my problems with sleep quality. But that is all behind me now. It is a working practice of mine now to get seven hours of sleep every night.

Good sleep influences the exquisite and vital balance of insulin, cortisol, and oxytocin. A mountain of evidence amassed by scientific researchers attests to the fact that too little sleep can raise insulin levels and lead to weight gain and insulin resistance. On the other hand, oxytocin released in the brain under stress-free conditions naturally promotes sleep, according to a 2003 study in the journal *Regulatory Peptides*. This makes sense because oxytocin has a calming effect. It leaves you feeling tranquil and loving, and certainly that helps your path to sleep.

Getting a good night's sleep resets our circadian rhythm, or internal body clock. There's a master circadian clock in the middle of the brain called the suprachiasmatic nuclei. It acts as a timekeeper for the rest of the body. Almost every hormone in your body is released according to this "clock." For example, it helps the body pump out the hormone melatonin when darkness falls—this tells the body when it's night, in turn helping us feel sleepy. Certain other hormones are more active long after the sun sets. Most of our growth hormone is released from the pituitary gland at the base of the brain during sleep—especially deep sleep, the most restorative stage of the sleep cycle. In adults, insufficient growth hormone is associated with fat formed around the tummy.

In women, follicle-stimulating hormone and luteinizing hormone—which regulate the function of the ovaries and control the reproductive system—are released at night too. FSH and LH decline during menopause, which is one reason why menopausal women notice more hot flashes and sweating at night.

How does your clock get properly "set"? It involves more than buying the right mattress or avoiding caffeine prior to bedtime (though both are important). More than anything, it has a lot to do with your eyes detecting light and dark. When your eyes detect light, this tells your brain (the hypothalamus, in particular) to wake up and release cortisol and other hormones you need to increase your metabolism and get through your day. When your eyes detect the colors of sunset and darkness, this tells your brain to release sleep hormones and wind down.

One of the best ways to keep your internal clock properly set is to catch sunrises and sunsets. The first thing I do in the morning is look out at the sunshine and let the light hit my eyes. In our house we also try to catch the sunsets. Sunsets naturally signal to our body that it is time to produce melatonin (our body's sleep hormone), that it's time to rest.

When you get proper sleep, your body gets an all-important time to rest and ready itself for a new day. Many wonderful things ensue: Your skin regenerates. Your blood pressure drops and vital functions, such as the beating of your heart, rate of your breathing, and urine output, reach their lowest points during sleep. Once you go to bed, your gut starts to slow at midnight, and then your liver begins to focus on housekeeping tasks, such as liberating calories to energize your vital organs.

Parts of the brain are more active during sleep. During the day, masses of information flood your brain, which temporarily stores it. But at night, during sleep, your brain converts these experiences into memory.

Research suggests the brain may also use sleep to cleanse toxins. A 2013 study published in the journal *Science* showed that brain cells temporarily shrink during sleep, opening gaps between the nerve cells that allow fluid to wash the brain clean. Interruptions to this process could contribute to diseases such as Parkinson's and Alzheimer's.

Here are ways to safeguard your needed beauty sleep:

Establish a healthy morning ritual. Think of it this way: A good evening starts with a good morning. A healthy morning routine will look different for every woman, but I enjoy gratitude journaling in the morning because it starts my day off by highlighting what I am grateful for and allowing me to set positive intentions for the rest of the day. I sip my Keto Coffee with breakfast, which is often a green smoothie. I might also take a short walk on the lawn or beach to ground with the Earth's natural energy. As mentioned, this gives me a chance to catch the sunrise.

Commit to Keto-Green fasting. Go at least thirteen to fifteen hours overnight, while sleeping, without food. Eating late can interfere with digestion. If you have food during the night, the digestion process slows down. The passage of food through your gastrointestinal tract is slower, and activity of the enzymes that break down food is hindered. All of this can cause constipation, digestive issues, heartburn, and tummyaches. Also, you don't want to go to bed on a full stomach. This can cause heartburn in some people. Leave at least three hours after your evening meal before sleeping.

Enjoy breakfast. It really is the most important meal. What we break our fast with sets the tone for the day, so be sure to have healthy protein and fats, but very low carbs, to keep insulin and ghrelin hormones low.

Get key lab work done. Low magnesium levels, which can be detected in bloodwork, can negatively impact your sleep. Make sure you are getting red blood cell (not serum) magnesium checked. Other markers to look for are low DHEA and IGF-1 levels. Also, if you have food allergies or food intolerances, these can impact your sleep. Talk with your doctor about testing and do an elimination diet to determine if you have food intolerance issues.

Try natural sleep aids. I routinely recommend a number of supplements to clients who suffer from insomnia, hormone imbalances, or mood issues. One of my favorites is bioidentical progesterone, applied as a cream or taken orally. Progesterone produces metabolites that work on sleep. You should see an immediate improvement in sleep, mood, and other symptoms. Oftentimes, improving sleep leads to changes in other body systems due to increased hormonal healing. You might also find that you are dreaming for the first time in a long time—a sign of restorative sleep.

I also recommend supplementing with 5-hydroxytryptophan (5-HTP). When we eat foods that contain the amino acid tryptophan, the body converts the tryptophan into 5-HTP, which is then converted into serotonin and then into melatonin. Higher melatonin levels dictate better depth and quality of sleep. 5-HTP is best taken on an empty stomach prior to bedtime. Typical dosages of 5-HTP can be from 50 to 200 milligrams. Take it with vitamin B6 for best results.

Additionally, you can take 1 to 3 milligrams of melatonin, preferably in the early to midevening, around sunset. Most people find that works better than at bedtime.

Turn off electronics by 9:00 P.M. (or, preferably, by sunset). Staring at computer and smartphone screens well into the night can disrupt your circadian rhythm, melatonin production, and thus your sleep. At times when I can't avoid doing this, I use an app on my computer called f.lux, which at least reduces the blue light on my screen at a certain preprogrammed time. This is important because blue light tells our eyes that it isn't nighttime, so then our body doesn't produce melatonin. You can also purchase blue-light-blocking eyeglasses (see dranna.com/resources) as well as blue-light-blocking screens for iPhones (try products from Zen Tech), and keep your phones and digital clocks in the bathroom (to block out any LED lights and reduce EMF exposure).

Stop the stimulants. Caffeine, sugar, and alcohol taken in the evening will keep you awake. Although alcoholic beverages can make you feel sleepy initially, alcohol ultimately disrupts sleep cycles, especially REM (dreaming) sleep—the type that helps refresh our bodies.

Create an environment conducive to sleep. Your bedroom is your "sleep haven." Keep the temperature at a comfortable level. Research shows that a cool (65°F), pitch-dark room improves sleep and reduces hot flashes. Use your bedroom for sleeping and lovemaking rather than for watching TV or using your computer in bed. Decorate it with colors you find soothing. Finally, keep your bedroom free of clutter so that it is a true place of rest and you can relax when you slip into bed. Clutter increases stress by provoking feelings of being overwhelmed and crowded. Decluttering creates a calm, serene setting and gives you a sense of peace and control.

Establish a healthy nighttime ritual. This might involve calming activities like a warm bath with lavender essential oils, sipping some chamomile or nighttime herbal tea, reading, or listening to music to make it easier to fall asleep. Light stretching will ease strain on your muscles and allow them to relax. Meditation and deep breathing help keep your hormones flowing naturally and support your natural rhythms.

My evening ritual often looks like this: I turn my bedroom temperature down to 65°F (or as close as I can get in summer without driving up my electric bill too much, typically 69°F), catch the sunset, go for a walk, and then stretch. I supplement with magnesium L-threonate (my Better Brain & Sleep formula), 3 milligrams of melatonin sublingual, and progesterone/pregnenolone cream (my Pura Balance PPr). I like a hot cup of tea, but I try not to drink after dinner, both to let my digestion work better and so that I won't get up in the middle of the night to use the bathroom. Then it's book and prayer time with my youngest daughter. I enjoy every minute of it.

Chapter 11

Master Your Most Important Hormone, Oxytocin

Throughout this book I've tried to explain the intricate dance that your hormones are constantly doing in your body and the ways in which hormonal imbalance leads to a wide array of uncomfortable physical symptoms as well as emotional discontent. The bottom line is that *your physiology drives your behavior*. To be more precise, your body's production of oxytocin, the hormone that enables bonding, closeness, and collaboration, plays a huge role in affecting your actions, your thoughts, and your feelings. It is your most important hormone. Cortisol is involved in driving behavior too, particularly if it is waging war with oxytocin. Cortisol keeps you stressed, while oxytocin keeps you calm. If cortisol wins the battle, you are prone to feeling irritable, fatigued, unfocused, and frustrated; your life feels chaotic. The balance between these two hormones and their interactions with our neural system give us feelings of connection or disconnection. So of course you want your oxytocin levels high. It is, in my opinion, our most powerful and healing hormone. It deserves a chapter all its own.

If you don't fix deficiencies of oxytocin, there can be consequences, some of them very severe. In fact, low levels of oxytocin are associated with several mental health conditions, including depression, anxiety, severe shyness (social phobia), autism, schizophrenia, PTSD, anorexia nervosa, and borderline personality disorder. Unfortunately, most conditions like these are treated with an arsenal of prescription mood drugs, which do not do much more than mask the symptoms.

Fortunately, you don't need an antidepressant, a tranquilizer, or a hormone pill. You just need to create more oxytocin in your life. The Hormone Fix will repair the emotional symptoms that are hurting your relationships and, indeed, your entire life.

When you boost oxytocin naturally, there are enormous benefits. As shown in many scientific studies, oxytocin:

- Enhances your sense of optimism, trust, mastery, and self-esteem
- Establishes intimacy and attachment
- Creates sexual arousal
- Helps women get through labor by stimulating uterine contractions
- Helps people overcome social inhibitions and fears
- Heals wounds (through its anti-inflammatory properties) and can relieve pain
- May be responsible for a series of beneficial metabolic effects that help weight loss
- Decreases health-damaging inflammation
- Strengthens memory
- Inhibits the development of tolerance to various addictive drugs in animal studies (opiates, cocaine, alcohol), and reduces withdrawal symptoms
- Has the potential to help people with depression and anxiety
- Reduces stress
- Increases generosity

It's clear that we really wouldn't be human without oxytocin—we would not possess the ability to be the social, caring men and women that we are.

To help explain how oxytocin-influenced physiology drives connection, let me introduce you to Rachel, who was forty-two when she came to see me. Although she appeared to be in great physical health and was fit, beautiful, and intelligent, she was distressed about her relationships and mood. She described herself as feeling "numb" and "detached."

To help her, I needed her full story, even events from the very beginning of her life. I learned that her mother had not been happy about being pregnant and may have had a difficult pregnancy. Both her parents were drug-addicted and emotionally distant. The family moved frequently. There was no extended family or nurturing relationships in her early youth.

Rachel's father abandoned the family when she was eight. Fortunately, her mom went into rehab, recovered, got a job, found a good church community, and made a stable home. Rachel excelled in school and college. She married young, at twenty-one, but the relationship ended after two years. She remarried several years later but struggled to stay in love and in monogamy. These were years of partying, heavy shopping, and casual flings.

When we met, Rachel had finalized her second divorce and was starting to do "interior" work—focusing on her emotional problems and her spiritual emptiness. I pointed out to her what to me was blaringly obvious: her "oxytocin-seeking behavior," as I call it. I explained to her about the oxytocin-cortisol connection and how oxytocin is lower in adults who experienced a lack of nurturing as a child or adverse childhood experiences. She was in essence self-medicating with sex, binge shopping, partying, and gift giving, all of which produce oxytocin but for her had negative consequences emotionally and financially.

Understanding how her physiology was driving her behavior, her actions, and her thoughts was the aha moment for her. She got it immediately and said, "In that case, I will use my behavior to healthfully drive my physiology."

Rachel learned how to create more oxytocin in her life in other ways and be in love in the present moment, finding joy in her daily life. When urges threatened to lead her off her life course, she would recognize those immediately and, with self-discipline and practice, choose differently. She is now happily remarried and starting a family. All of these actions and choices help build oxytocin.

Thankfully, there are fun, natural ways to boost oxytocin that you've probably not heard much about before. I've got some amazing oxytocin fixes that you can start using right away.

The Oxytocin-Orgasm Connection

An orgasm is the number one way to produce more oxytocin—so I want to make sure you understand what actually happens during one and, more important, to make sure that you're having plenty of them. But first it's important to understand how a woman's orgasm is different from a man's, and to appreciate the good news that sexual intimacy without an actual orgasm still counts toward reaping the physical benefits of orgasm.

For many years—indeed, since 1966, when the groundbreaking book *Human Sexual Response*, by William Masters and Virginia Johnson, was first published—sex researchers had accepted the existence of a linear sexual response for both men and women: excitement/arousal, plateau, orgasm, and resolution. But over the past decade, the veracity of this model for everyone has come into question.

A man's sexual response does indeed follow those stages. He gets excited, builds to an orgasm, and then it's over—a crescendo that is goal-oriented. His goal is to climax. Most men also have the goal of getting you to climax; if you don't, a man may think it's the result of a bad performance on his part, and if you do, he gives himself a "bravo."

As you might be able to attest, though, women do not always move progressively and sequentially through these stages. Desire and sexual response for women are different. Researchers now accept that for most women, the process is more circuitous, not so linear and goal-oriented. Sometimes you start because you feel sexually excited. But sometimes you start because you're open to the idea. Indeed, many women may rarely or never want to initiate sex, but once they get started they get turned on. This is called secondary desire, and it is absolutely natural. That's why it can help to stop saying "I'm not feeling it" and instead say "Let me see how I'm going to feel." Starting from a place of willingness is perfectly fine. As you kiss, caress, and get turned on physically, along comes arousal.

I liken a man's direct arousal to driving on the highway: fast and aiming for the destination. For women, it is more like taking the scenic route, including sometimes stopping on the side of the road to take pictures or look at the view. In my Sexual CPR online education program, I make the analogy to the game Candyland. Sometimes you get stuck and go back a few steps, and sometimes you score candy, but in the end, it is all fun and good. I prefer to redefine orgasm as the entire journey and experience, with the climax as the cherry on top, so to speak.

All throughout lovemaking, whenever we feel pleasure, we're producing oxytocin. It's not just when we have physical satisfaction (the orgasm) but also when we experience emotional satisfaction (a feeling of intimacy and connection with a partner).

When we feel good about this pleasure, the sexual experience can be heightened. But quite often our partner presses us to climax as a measure of our pleasure and his success. So we really do need to tell our partner what it is we want. You could start by saying to your partner, "I love being sexual with you, but sex for me is not just intercourse. It's the lead-up." Or you could tell him: "For five minutes, let's do nothing else but caress."

During foreplay, you may start to feel sexy and warm as the blood starts to head toward your vagina and clitoris. More lubrication occurs in the walls of your vagina. As more blood flows to your pelvic area, muscle tension starts to build in your pelvis, buttocks, genitals, and thighs. Your breathing speeds up. Your nipples may become erect, and your heart rate increases.

As many as thirty areas of your brain play a role during this period of sexual arousal. Your orbitofrontal cortex, for example, which is involved in behavior control, temporarily shuts down, and your inhibitions sometimes disappear. Also, parts of your brain are flooded with oxytocin at this time. This makes you feel loved, connected, and bonded with your partner. There is an increase in feel-good endorphins that are naturally calming and mood-enhancing. If and when you climax, more oxytocin is secreted, and your vagina begins to contract. At the same time, your uterus acts like a suction cup. This is by design—to let sperm come in after ejaculation. It is nature's way of helping with conception.

When I speak of a woman's orgasm, as I've noted, I am talking about the entire sexual experience. It doesn't have to be about whether or not you were able to climax, because through the entire lovemaking session, you're producing oxytocin, and that is a win—that is, if you are present during the experience and not just going through the motions.

Intimacy strengthens your relationship with your partner; it is what gives you pleasure and enjoyment. Following your intimate moments, it is important to stay present—talking, holding each other, laughing, and just sharing in the intimacy before separating (or going to sleep). (I also offer a webinar, "Help, Doctor, My Sex Drive Has No Pulse!"; see dranna. com/resources.)

HEALTH BENEFITS OF INTIMACY AND ORGASM

- Pain relief. Oxytocin released during intimacy and orgasm helps to decrease pain sensations, particularly the pain associated with chronic menstrual cramping, migraines, dysmenorrhea, and endometriosis. Research has shown that orgasm decreases the sensation of pain up to 70 percent in women with fibromyalgia—better results than you'd get from taking an over-the-counter pain reliever. That excuse of "I have a headache" just won't work, because a nice climax eliminates that pain!
- Cardiovascular health. Oxytocin is produced mainly in the hypothalamus, but it is synthesized and has receptors in the heart too. This means that orgasms also benefit our cardiovascular system. There is even evidence that frequent orgasms may protect against heart attacks. As a form of exercise, sex helps the cardiac muscles and reduces the body's blood pressure in the long run and the risk of heart attacks.
- Brain fitness. MRI images show that women's brains utilize much more oxygen during orgasm than usual, similar to the effects of exercise. In other words, the

brain is being nourished, which helps keep your mind sharp. Orgasms also increase the hormone DHEA, which improves memory and brain function.

- Mood boost. Orgasm relieves anxiety and depression because oxytocin and other feel-good hormones such as serotonin are released, while cortisol is suppressed. Orgasms serve as a relaxant and give an overall good feeling. Oxytocin counteracts depression by flushing the system with endorphins (feel-good hormones).

- Incontinence control. Orgasms strengthen your pelvic muscles, and therefore improve bladder control.

- Libido lift. A hormone normally associated with men, testosterone helps boost sex drive in women. During an orgasm, and in general, oxytocin elevates estrogen and testosterone levels in the body, boosting sexual desire. The ovaries (in women) and testes (in men) also produce oxytocin.

- Better sleep. As mentioned, endorphins, our feel-good hormones, are released with orgasm. This produces an increased sense of relaxation, satisfaction, and desire for sleep.

- Appetite control. Orgasms can reduce your appetite and cravings. Throughout sexual activity, the body produces phenylethylamine—a natural amphetamine that can help to lessen cravings for junk food and cigarettes. Orgasm and intimacy also make you feel like your emotional needs have been met, so you're less likely to dive into ice cream or french fries for comfort. Pleasure is your "comfort food"!

- Stronger immunity. According to researchers at Wilkes University in Pennsylvania, people who have regular sex have higher levels of immunoglobulin A, or IgA, an important antibody that fends off infection. Another study shows that women who report enjoying sexual activity live longer than do women who reported less pleasure in sex. One reason for the longevity bonus could be that orgasms have positive effects on various organs and body systems. Studies indicate that as sexual activity goes up, the risk of breast cancer goes down. This could be due to the surge of hormones such as oxytocin that comes with arousal and orgasm. Oxytocin reduces disease-causing free radicals in the body. Free radicals can cause DNA damage and activate pro-carcinogens, which can become carcinogens (substances capable of causing cancer).

Other Ways to Increase Oxytocin

Fortunately, there are other activities besides sex that cause the release of oxytocin, all of them fun and pleasurable. These will bring about bonding between you and others, as well as helping you feel more optimistic and happy and strengthen your sense of well-being.

- Cuddle on the couch with your loved one during a mushy feel-good movie—a certified oxytocin-boosting move. A study at the University of North Carolina at Chapel Hill found that women who snuggled with their mate during a romantic video experienced a surge of oxytocin. Cuddling with your kids increases oxytocin too, as does a head rub or massage.
- Hug frequently. A loving hug can help break the ice between strangers, strengthen bonds between friends, and dissolve bitterness between enemies. It eases our tension, fear, and anxiety at tough moments when we feel stressed. Notice how your body feels after receiving the hug or caress. Does it feel warmer, softer, calmer? That's the effect of surging oxytocin. It is amazing how one simple hug can change your biochemical experience.

- Try self-hugging, self-caressing, and self-pleasuring. Hugging yourself might seem a bit silly at first, but your body doesn't register that. It simply reacts to the physical feeling of warmth and care, just as a baby responds to being cradled in its mother's arms. Physical touch has the power to release oxytocin, reduce cortisol, and calm stress. So why not try it? Whenever you're feeling stressed, upset, or self-critical, give yourself a hug. Make it a habit—a clear gesture that conveys feelings of love, care, and tenderness. Lovingly touch your body in the shower while washing. Give yourself positive affirmations about the physical masterpiece that is you.
- Heat up. Oxytocin is commonly activated by warm temperatures. Researchers have found that warm environments and increased sweating activate specific oxytocin-producing parts of the hypothalamus, just as breastfeeding does in mother and infant. Try a sauna, a steambath, or a hot yoga session, or bask in sunlight. Exercise also increases oxytocin, and this may be why I am always happier leaving the gym than going to it!
- Socialize. The body churns out oxytocin when you're in large social gatherings. This happens naturally to help achieve more harmony and oneness among the group. Do you know what the most oxytocin-rich environment is? You guessed it—a wedding, with the bride releasing the most and the mother of the bride a close second!

  Researchers have found that your brain releases more oxytocin during social contact and social bonding, and this can actually speed up healing from disease. In the cultures around the world in which people are the longest-lived (often called "blue zones"), people have strong community ties. In community, we give and receive, and this increases oxytocin. So my advice is to participate in community activities, your church, and outreach to others.
- Nurture your friendships. A propensity for healing relationships seems to be part of female genetic wiring; it is inherently related to oxytocin, which is released when women interact socially. Whatever the reason, women need other women—we guide each

other, console each other, and celebrate with each other. The long-running Harvard-based Nurses' Health Study found that the more close friends a woman has, the less likely she is to suffer physical ills as she ages. In fact, not having at least one true confidante can ultimately be as detrimental to your health as being a heavy smoker! And sharing emotions with good pals also soothes frazzled nerves. All of this points to the release of oxytocin when we bond with others. In fact, UCLA researchers report that women release oxytocin when stressed, which generates an urge to "bond"—yet once that urge is satisfied, we produce even more oxytocin, ultimately creating a calming sensation. You've probably heard that an occasional glass of red wine can improve longevity because it contains resveratrol, a powerful antioxidant. I always emphasize that having wine in the company of friends, family, and laughter might actually be what makes the wine so good for you.

- Care for a pet. When you interact with animals, researchers find, you have increased levels of oxytocin. A review of sixty-nine studies on human-animal interactions showed that contact with animals, especially your own pet, increases oxytocin production, which counters elevated levels of stress and anxiety. The results also suggested that while single meetings with animals trigger the oxytocin effects, stable relationships, like pet ownership or at least regular interactions, are linked to more potent and longer-lasting effects.

- Be generous. Giving is a way to increase oxytocin. Just try it and see. I regularly volunteer at church with the kids' groups. I also created a foundation in honor of my son, called the Garrett V. Bivens Foundation. Through it, we've done some very beautiful things, including teaching-tots-to-swim programs and helping to found the House of Hope, a safe home and rehabilitation center for girls who've been caught up in human trafficking.

- Try acupuncture. In a 2013 review of the effects of acupuncture on the neuroendocrine system, this ancient Chinese practice has been shown to stimulate the release of endorphins and oxytocin, leading to the reduction of stress and pain.

NUTRIENTS AND HERBS THAT INCREASE OXYTOCIN

Going Keto-Green in both diet and lifestyle will help reestablish your circadian rhythm and normalize your cortisol production and response. These actions help tremendously for improving levels of oxytocin. Several of the supplements I suggest you take on the ten-day Quick Start and subsequent twenty-one-day (or lifelong) diet will also help restore and encourage oxytocin release.

Vitamin C

Vitamin C is an easy way to optimize and increase your levels of oxytocin. One 2002 German study found that vitamin C stimulated the secretion of oxytocin, increased frequency of sexual activity, improved mood, and reduced stress.

As you may know, vitamin C is found in vegetables and fruits such as green peppers, citrus fruits, tomatoes, cauliflower, and cabbage—all good alkalinizing foods too.

Vitamin D

Vitamin D is actually technically a hormone, not a vitamin. Research shows that serotonin, oxytocin, and vasopressin—three brain hormones that affect social behavior—are all activated by vitamin D. Some researchers believe that autistic children have low levels of oxytocin because they are likely deficient in vitamin D.

Ideally, you should get your vitamin D from the sun, but you can also obtain it through supplementation.

Magnesium

I've covered this amazing mineral throughout this book. It's perhaps the most important mineral in your body, yet most people don't know that oxytocin receptors on cells require magnesium to function properly. Plus, most people are deficient in this nutrient. Is it any wonder that so many of us feel disconnected and out of sorts?

There are a number of ways you can increase magnesium in your body. First, make sure you're eating magnesium-rich foods on a regular basis: spinach, chard, pumpkin seeds, almonds, and avocado. These foods are included on my Keto-Green Diet.

Also, you can take a multivitamin-mineral supplement that contains magnesium as insurance. My choices are magnesium malate, magnesium lysinate glycinate chelate, and magnesium L-threonate because they can cross the protective blood-brain barrier and thus work better in the body and brain. You can also consider trying transdermal (topical) magnesium. When you apply magnesium on your skin, your body will absorb the amount it needs.

Methylators

Methylation is a process that transforms toxins into safer substances in the body. It also supports the oxytocin receptors on cells that open up and let this hormone in. This process depends on a number of nutrients, including folate, vitamin B6, and vitamin B12, so it is worth supplementing with a B complex vitamin. See the Resources section for multivitamin recommendations.

Chamomile

Chamomile tea has been used for centuries in the Roman Empire, during Egyptian rule, and in ancient Greece. Prized for its many phytochemicals, chamomile offers numerous calming, anti-inflammatory, and health-boosting benefits. Researchers have also discovered that chamomile naturally increases oxytocin and lowers cortisol. I recommend chamomile tea on my diet. Chamomile essential oils can also be enjoyed regularly.

Melatonin

Melatonin is a hormone released by your pineal gland, a tiny gland in your brain. It helps control your sleep-wake cycle (your circadian rhythm). Adequate levels of melatonin are necessary to fall asleep quickly and sleep deeply through the night. Many scientific studies have shown that 500 micrograms (0.5 milligram) of melatonin daily can significantly increase the production of oxytocin.

Oxytocin and Self-Compassion

Practice self-compassion at all times—being good and kind to yourself and not beating yourself up when you suffer, fail, or feel inadequate. When we soothe ourselves with the healing balm of self-compassion, not only are we changing our mental and emotional experience, we're also changing our body chemistry. Self-compassion triggers the release of oxytocin—and it's something you can practice and do all the time for a steady flow of this master hormone.

How exactly do you develop—and practice—self-compassion? In short, it involves having the same attitude toward yourself that you have toward a close friend. Rather than criticizing her, judging her, and adding to her stress, you listen with empathy and understanding. You encourage her to remember that mistakes are only normal, and validate her emotions without adding fuel to the fire. If you can talk to yourself as compassionately as you would to your best friend, you'll start to see yourself as someone with great value. And eventually you'll be able to tap into that self-loving mindset whenever you're in a tough spot.

Self-compassion, by definition, is the act of being less critical toward yourself. This is important. When we are harsh on ourselves, we activate the sympathetic nervous system (the fight-or-flight reaction) and elevate stress hormones such as cortisol in our bloodstream. Self-compassion, by contrast, releases oxytocin, allowing us to calmly evaluate a situation without attacking ourselves. A simple exercise is to look at yourself in the mirror, into your eyes, and speak loving truths to your precious self and do some positive coaching. Sometimes it is helpful to think of your earliest childhood self when you do this practice. Try saying: "You are so precious and just wonderfully created. You have the potential to do anything you really want to do. You are healthy, loving, kind, and good," and continue from there. You may feel self-conscious, but you'll also find that speaking kindly and encouragingly to yourself feels good; this is a powerful practice.

Epilogue

A Final Message

I believe every woman deserves a life filled with good health, happiness, and overflowing with love. With the right nutrition, an optimized lifestyle, and simple, loving actions, you can dramatically alter and balance your hormonal chemistry. I wrote this book especially for you. I want you to live the most beautiful and vibrant life that you absolutely can.

With our hormones fixed, and working for us, not against us, we become more resilient, getting up even when we would rather not, being loving when we'd rather hide, and being kind when we could be angry.

Our life is a journey that we traverse in our own unique ways and circumstances, but we are not alone. Be encouraged: You are joining a community of women who want a better life for themselves and their families. We have so much life to live and so much yet to give. I look forward to continuing this discovery process and successful path with you. You are worth it, and I believe in you!

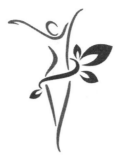

PART FOUR

· ·

Keto-Green Recipes

KETO-GREEN SMOOTHIES

DR. ANNA'S BASIC KETO-GREEN
SMOOTHIE

INGREDIENTS

> 1 scoop Dr. Anna's Keto-Alkaline Protein* Shake powder
> (0 g sugar)
> 1 tablespoon MCT or coconut oil
> 2 scoops Mighty Maca Plus
> 8 ounces water

DIRECTIONS

Place all ingredients in a shaker cup, NutriBullet, or blender and shake or blend until smooth. Delicious!

*Note: You can substitute a similar protein powder you love and do well with for my Keto-Alkaline Protein. Just be conscientious about making sure the macronutrient and micronutrient profiles are close to those of mine.

MAKES 1 SERVING

DR. ANNA'S FAVORITE
SUPER KETO-GREEN SMOOTHIE

INGREDIENTS

1 scoop Dr. Anna's Keto-Alkaline Protein Shake powder

1 tablespoon MCT or coconut oil

2 scoops Mighty Maca Plus

Handful of kale

1 stalk of celery

½-inch-thick slice of fresh ginger root

¼ avocado

Dash of cardamom or fresh mint

1 teaspoon each of chia seeds and flaxseed (or pumpkin and sunflower seeds)

8 ounces water with 3–4 cubes of ice

DIRECTIONS

Place all ingredients in a blender and blend until smooth. Delicious!

MAKES 1 SERVING

Optional: With my Basic Keto-Green Smoothie: Add in great-tasting alkaline additions for this smoothie (Choose one to a few of the below. Mix and match to come up with your own delicious recipes).

Fresh ginger

Avocado

1 tablespoon pumpkin, sunflower, or chia seeds, and/or freshly ground flaxseeds

Almond or cashew butter

Tamarind

Spinach and/or other greens

Mint

Cilantro

Collagen/protein powder

Cucumber

Celery

Coconut water, milk, or flakes

Cinnamon

Cardamom

Pomegranate

Vanilla extract

Ice cream (just kidding!)

DIRECTIONS

Place all ingredients in a blender and blend until smooth.

MAKES 1 SERVING

ISLAND GREEN SMOOTHIE

INGREDIENTS

1 cup mixed greens such as kale, spinach, collards, and so
forth

Juice of ½ lime

Fresh ginger root to taste, approximately ¼ inch, peeled and
chopped

¼ avocado

¼ cup unsweetened coconut flakes

1 tablespoon coconut or MCT oil

1½ cups water

1–2 tablespoons powdered maca (optional)

Greens (optional)

DIRECTIONS

Place all ingredients in a blender and blend until smooth.

MAKES 1 SERVING

CREAMY VANILLA MINT SMOOTHIE

INGREDIENTS

    1 cup baby spinach

    10–12 mint leaves

    1 tablespoon almond butter

    ¼ teaspoon vanilla extract

    1½ cups unsweetened almond milk or coconut milk

DIRECTIONS

Place all ingredients in a blender and blend until smooth.

MAKES 1 SERVING

LEMON GINGER ZINGER

INGREDIENTS

½ cup fresh dandelion greens

½ cup fresh spinach

1 2-inch piece of fresh ginger root, peeled and chopped

1 teaspoon lemon juice

¼ avocado

1½ cups water

1 scoop collagen protein powder

1–2 tablespoons powdered maca (optional) or scoops Mighty
Maca Plus (optional)

DIRECTIONS

Place all ingredients in a blender and blend until smooth.

MAKES 1 SERVING

NUTTY FOR GREEN SMOOTHIE

INGREDIENTS

1 cup fresh spinach

¼ avocado

8–10 cashews

1 tablespoon unsweetened coconut flakes

1 teaspoon cinnamon

1 cup cashew milk (or other nut milk)

1–2 tablespoons powdered maca (optional) or scoops Mighty
Maca Plus (optional)

DIRECTIONS

Place all ingredients in a blender and blend until smooth.

MAKES 1 SERVING

POWER-UP SMOOTHIE

INGREDIENTS

1 cucumber, chopped

1 stalk celery, chopped

¼ avocado

1 teaspoon spirulina or Mighty Maca Plus (optional)

1 teaspoon each of chia seeds and flaxseeds

1 tablespoon MCT oil

Thin slice of ginger root, peeled (optional)

1 cup water

3–4 ice cubes

DIRECTIONS

Place all ingredients in a blender and blend until smooth.

MAKES 1 SERVING

BREAKFASTS

COCONUT ALMOND PANCAKES

INGREDIENTS

1 cup almond flour

¼ cup unsweetened coconut flakes

½ teaspoon aluminum-free baking powder

Pinch sea salt

½ cup unsweetened almond milk

½ teaspoon pure vanilla extract

3 large organic cage-free eggs, beaten

1 tablespoon organic ghee

2–3 tablespoons almond butter

1–2 cups fresh berries, your choice

2 teaspoons maple syrup (optional)

2 tablespoons organic whipped cream (optional)

DIRECTIONS

Combine the almond flour, coconut flakes, baking powder, and salt in a large bowl.

Combine the almond milk, vanilla, and eggs in a separate bowl. Make a well in the dry ingredients and pour in the egg mixture, mixing well.

Heat a pan over medium heat, add the ghee, and swirl to coat the pan. Ladle a few spoonfuls of pancake batter into the pan and cook for 3 to 5 minutes. Flip and cook for another 2 to 4 minutes, until golden. Repeat, if needed, until all the batter is used.

Heat the almond butter until warm and drizzle a spoonful over each stack of pancakes along with the maple syrup, if using, and top with whipped cream, if desired. Garnish with berries and serve.

MAKES 2 SERVINGS

GREEN EGGS AND BACON

INGREDIENTS

2 tablespoons pesto (premade)

⅓ cup almonds

1 large bunch fresh basil

2 tablespoons fresh lemon juice

1 garlic clove, sliced

5 tablespoons extra-virgin olive oil

½ teaspoon coconut aminos (optional)

3 slices bacon

1 tablespoon organic ghee (or extra-virgin olive oil)

2 large organic cage-free eggs

⅓ medium avocado, sliced

DIRECTIONS

Blend together pesto, almonds, basil, lemon juice, garlic, oil, and coconut aminos in a food processor or blender. Season with salt. Set aside.

In a frying pan, fry the bacon until crisp, about 2 minutes per side. Set bacon aside.

In the same frying pan, over medium-low heat, crack the eggs into the pan and season with salt and pepper. If the oil starts to spit, it's too hot, so turn down the heat. Cook the eggs until the white is set and the yolk is still runny, or to your liking.

Place the eggs and bacon on a plate. Top with sliced avocado and 2 tablespoons pesto mixture. Store any remaining pesto mixture in the fridge (try it with a fresh salad or roast chicken).

MAKES 2 SERVINGS

KETO CHORIZO EGG MUFFINS

INGREDIENTS

3–5 ounces Spanish chorizo (or pancetta or pepperoni)
1 cup chopped kale
6 large organic cage-free eggs
½ cup grated cheddar cheese or goat cheese (optional)
Sriracha sauce (optional)
Greens (optional)
Sliced avocado (optional)

DIRECTIONS

Preheat the oven to 350°F.

Dice the chorizo and place into a hot dry pan. Cook for 1 to 2 minutes, until hot and crisped.

Add the kale to the chorizo and cook for another 5 minutes over medium-low heat until soft. Remove from the heat and set aside.

Crack the eggs into a bowl and beat. Add the chorizo and kale. Season with salt and pepper. Add the grated cheese (if using).

Divide the mixture evenly among 10 muffin cups (a silicone muffin pan works best), or pour the mixture into a skillet to make a frittata.

Bake for 20 to 25 minutes. Cool slightly before serving.

Serve with sriracha sauce, if desired, greens, and/or sliced avocado, if desired.

Store leftovers in the fridge in an airtight container for up to 5 days.

MAKES 5 SERVINGS

KETO OMELET WRAP

INGREDIENTS

    2 large organic cage-free eggs

    2 tablespoons organic cheese (optional)

    2 tablespoons chopped fresh chives

    1 tablespoon organic ghee

    4 ounces smoked salmon, thinly sliced

    ½ avocado, sliced

    1 medium scallion, chopped

DIRECTIONS

Crack the eggs into a bowl and season with salt and pepper and beat well with a whisk or fork.

In a small bowl, mix the cheese (if using) with chopped chives. Set aside.

Heat a pan over medium heat and add the ghee. Pour the eggs into the pan and cook, using a spatula to bring in the egg from the sides toward the center for the first 30 seconds, for 1 to 2 minutes. Be sure not to overcook. Add in the cheese (optional) and chives.

Slide the omelet onto a plate. Top with the salmon, avocado, and scallion, and fold into a wrap.

MAKES 2 SERVINGS

EGGS BENEDICT WITH SMOKED SALMON AND SPINACH

INGREDIENTS

2 cups fresh chopped spinach, tightly packed

4 ounces smoked salmon, thinly sliced

4 large organic free-range eggs

1 large tomato

½ cup Hollandaise sauce (recipe follows)

DIRECTIONS

In a saucepan, cook the spinach, drain well, and return it to the pan. Place the salmon in the pan next to the spinach.

Use an egg poacher to poach the eggs according to the manufacturer's directions. If you don't have an egg poacher, add enough water to two medium saucepans to fill them about 2 inches deep. Add 1 teaspoon salt and 2 teaspoons vinegar to each pan and bring to a gentle simmer. Crack 2 eggs into two separate small bowls, keeping the yolks intact. When the water is simmering, use the handle of a spatula or spoon to quickly stir the water (one pan at a time) in one direction until the water is swirling in the pan. Gently drop 1 egg at a time into the center of the whirlpool in each pan. The swirling water will help prevent the white from feathering or spreading out in the pan. Cover and let the eggs poach, setting your timer for 5 minutes; leave the eggs untouched while poaching. Repeat for the second serving of eggs.

While the eggs are poaching, gently warm the spinach, smoked salmon, and Hollandaise sauce. Put one thick tomato slice on each of two plates.

Divide the warm spinach between the two plates. Top each with half the salmon.

When the eggs are ready, remove them from the water with a slotted spoon, place two poached eggs on top of the spinach and salmon, and drizzle with Hollandaise.

MAKES 2 SERVINGS

HOLLANDAISE SAUCE

INGREDIENTS

 3 egg yolks
 1 tablespoon lemon juice
 Cayenne pepper
 ½ stick organic butter, melted

DIRECTIONS

 Blend the egg yolks and juice with a whisk or fork. Season with salt, pepper, and cayenne.

 Slowly add the melted butter so as not to break the sauce, whisking continuously.

MAKES 2 SERVINGS

KETO-COCONUT YOGURT BERRY BOWL

INGREDIENTS

> 1 cup organic plain yogurt or dairy-free yogurt
> ½ cup fresh berries
> 1 cup chopped nuts, any type
> 1 tablespoon chia seeds
> 1–2 teaspoons xylitol, monk fruit, or stevia, to taste
> 1–2 tablespoons unsweetened shredded coconut

DIRECTIONS

Combine all the ingredients in a bowl. Top with a dash of ground cinnamon, if desired.

MAKES 2 SERVINGS

KETO SLOW-COOKER BREAKFAST CASSEROLE

INGREDIENTS

3 slices bacon

½ cup chopped red bell pepper

1 cup chopped mushrooms

3 tablespoons chopped shallots or onions

8 large leaves of kale, finely shredded

8 large organic cage-free eggs

1 tablespoon organic butter or ghee

½ to 1 cup shredded Parmesan cheese or cheese of choice (optional)

DIRECTIONS

Cook the bacon until almost crisp. Add the red peppers, mushrooms, and shallots or onions. Sauté until the vegetables are softened and the bacon is crisp.

Add the kale and turn off the heat to allow it to wilt but not overcook.

In a bowl, beat the eggs. Season with salt and pepper.

Turn a slow cooker on high and place the butter in to melt. Once melted, brush the inside of the slow cooker with the melted butter.

Place the sautéed vegetable mixture into the base of the slow cooker.

Sprinkle the cheese over the vegetables, if using, and then pour the egg mixture on top.

Stir and cook on high for approximately 1½ hours, or on low for about 6 hours. These times can vary depending on your slow cooker.

If desired, serve with spinach and sliced avocado dressed with extra-virgin olive oil.

MAKES 4 SERVINGS

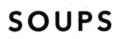

SOUPS

BONE BROTH

INGREDIENTS

2 unpeeled carrots, scrubbed and roughly chopped

2 stalks celery, including leafy part, roughly chopped

1 medium onion, roughly chopped

7 cloves garlic, peeled and smashed

3½ pounds grass-fed beef bones (preferably joints and knuckles)

2 bay leaves

2 teaspoons sea salt

2 tablespoons apple cider vinegar

DIRECTIONS

Place all the ingredients into a slow cooker. Add water to cover by 1 inch. Cook on low for 8 to 10 hours.

Use a shallow spoon to carefully skim any film off the top of the broth. Pour the broth through a fine-mesh strainer and discard the solids. Taste the broth and add salt as needed. The broth will keep for 3 days in the fridge and 3 months in the freezer.

Variations: Feel free to substitute chicken, fish, or pork bones, or to combine them all. Also, try adding dried mushrooms or 2 tablespoons fish sauce in place of the salt to dramatically boost the flavor of the broth.

ALKALINE BROTH*

INGREDIENTS

2 unpeeled carrots, scrubbed and roughly chopped

2 stalks celery, including leafy part, roughly chopped

1 medium onion, roughly chopped

7 cloves garlic, peeled and smashed

1 cup cauliflower or broccoli florets

2 bay leaves

2 teaspoons sea salt

2 tablespoons apple cider vinegar

Optional: Add vegetable remnants from your week's food preps. I love to save the stems and extra leaves for my bone broth or alkaline broth.

DIRECTIONS

Place all the ingredients in a slow cooker. Add water to cover by 1 inch. Cook on low for 8 to 10 hours.

(Or place in a pressure cooker or InstaPot and cook for 60 minutes on high.)

*You can substitute this for Bone Broth anytime.

EASY TOMATO SOUP

INGREDIENTS

 3 tablespoons extra-virgin olive oil
 1 medium yellow onion, diced
 2 large cloves garlic, minced
 1 large stalk celery, diced
 1 teaspoon sea salt
 2 (28-ounce) cans Italian plum tomatoes, diced or crushed
 12 ounces bone broth

DIRECTIONS

Heat olive oil in a saucepan on medium heat. Add onion, garlic, celery, and salt. Sauté for 5 minutes.

Add tomatoes and broth. Bring to a boil over high heat, then reduce heat and simmer for 10 minutes. Add pepper and more salt to taste.

For a creamier, more refined soup, use an immersion blender to puree the soup right in the saucepan.

Swirl in a little more olive oil just before serving, if desired. You can garnish with your favorite chopped fresh herbs—basil, thyme, flat-leaf (Italian) parsley, and so forth.

MAKES 4 SERVINGS

THAI COCONUT SOUP

INGREDIENTS

1 whole organic or pasture-raised chicken (about 4 pounds)

2 teaspoons sea salt

6 stalks lemongrass, sliced in half lengthwise and then in thirds

2 inches fresh ginger root, peeled and sliced thinly

8 Kaffir lime leaves (optional)

2 yellow or white onions, diced (about 5 cups)

4 stalks celery, sliced into 1-inch slices (about 2 cups)

4 carrots, peeled and sliced into 1-inch rounds (about 2 cups)

1 cup sliced crimini or shiitake mushrooms

½ cup sliced bamboo shoots

1 cup sliced baby zucchini

1 cup snap or snow peas (optional)

½ can organic coconut milk

1 cup freshly squeezed lime juice (from 4–8 limes)

2 tablespoons fish sauce (optional)

Cilantro, chopped (optional)

DIRECTIONS

Place chicken in a large pot; add salt and cover with water. Bring to a boil. Skim off any solids that float to the surface. Reduce to a simmer.

Add lemongrass, ginger, and lime leaves (if using). Simmer on low for 2 to 3 hours until chicken is tender and falling apart.

Remove chicken from pot and place on platter or bowl. Set aside.

Add onions, celery, and carrots to the pot and simmer for about 15 to 20 minutes, or until tender. Turn off heat. Add mushrooms, bamboo shoots, and zucchini. Add snap or snow peas if using.

When chicken is cool enough to handle, remove meat from the bones, shred, and add back into the pot. (Reserve bones for future broth making.)

Stir in coconut milk and lime juice. Add fish sauce if using. Salt, to taste. Garnish with cilantro, if using.

Note: You can also adapt this recipe to make in a pressure cooker or slow cooker. Leftover soup is great to have on hand. It will last in the fridge for five days in a sealed container.

MAKES 4 SERVINGS

SOUP AND SANDWICH, ANYONE?

You can easily build your own Keto-Green Sandwich using a Keto-Green wrap such as nori sheets or large leaf lettuce (romaine and Bibb lettuce are two of my favorites).

Begin by layering on your protein. Examples include sardines, smoked salmon, chicken, tuna, or some nitrate-free lunch meat.

Add some greens, along with some sliced onions, salt, pepper, extra-virgin olive oil, or sriracha mayo (sriracha sauce mixed with a little mayonnaise). Consider adding in some broccoli sprouts for additional crunch and nutritional boost. Wrap it up and enjoy.

SALADS

SPINACH AND KALE SALAD WITH BACON AND CHICKEN

INGREDIENTS

4 slices bacon

1 medium onion, thinly sliced

1 pound organic or pasture-raised chicken breasts, cubed

½ cup sliced mushrooms

1 bunch each of baby spinach and kale (4 packed cups)

2 tablespoons Basil Thyme Vinaigrette (recipe on page 251)

Sprouts, chopped parsley, and sunflower seeds, for garnish

DIRECTIONS

Place the bacon in a pan over medium heat and cook for 5 minutes, until slightly crisp. Set the bacon aside and drain half of the fat from the pan.

Add the onion and ¼ teaspoon salt to the remaining fat in the pan and cook over medium-low heat for 20 minutes, stirring occasionally.

Increase the heat to medium high. Add the chicken and mushrooms, and continue to cook for 8 minutes, or until the chicken is cooked through.

Roughly chop the bacon, then return it to the pan just long enough to reheat it. Remove the skillet from the heat.

Place the spinach and kale in a bowl. Add the vinaigrette and toss. Spoon the hot chicken mixture over the spinach. Top with sprouts, parsley, and sunflower seeds.

MAKES 4 SERVINGS

BRUSSELS SPROUTS–KALE SALAD BOWL

INGREDIENTS

1 tablespoon minced shallots

2 garlic cloves, minced

2 tablespoons Dijon mustard

¼ cup fresh lemon juice

¼ cup extra-virgin olive oil

8 mint leaves, finely chopped

1 large bunch kale

15 Brussels sprouts

1 bunch parsley, leaves finely chopped

⅓ cup raw almonds, chopped

2 tablespoons pine nuts

1 tablespoon pomegranate seeds

DIRECTIONS

For the dressing, combine shallots, garlic, mustard, lemon juice, oil, and mint in a bowl. Whisk to combine. Set aside.

Prepare the kale by washing and removing the thick stems. Next, roll the leaves and slice to create thin strips.

Prepare the Brussels sprouts by chopping off the thick stalk, cutting each in half, and slicing very finely. I use a VeggieBullet or food processor during my weekly food prep for simplicity.

Place the kale, Brussels sprouts, parsley, and almonds in a bowl and toss well. Add the pine nuts, pomegranate seeds, and dressing. Toss again. (The kale and Brussels sprouts can also be roasted or sautéed first to make a warm salad, which is my preference in the winter months.)

Variation: Add avocado and bacon.

MAKES 2 TO 4 SERVINGS

SPRING COBB SALAD

INGREDIENTS

1 head lettuce (romaine or butter) or escarole, torn, or
   1 bunch watercress

Dressing of choice, enough to coat salad (see page 249)

1 pound organic roasted turkey breast, cubed or cut into
   strips

8 slices bacon, cooked and crumbled

4 hard-boiled large organic cage-free eggs, diced

1 avocado, diced

4 radishes, halved and sliced

1 cup celery, diced

1 cup sprouts

DIRECTIONS

In a large bowl, toss the lettuce with dressing. Place the dressed greens on a large serving dish.

Place the turkey on top, forming a row down the middle. In strips on either side of the turkey, place the remaining ingredients. Drizzle with additional dressing, if desired.

MAKES 4 SERVINGS

BROCCOLI SLAW AND EGG SALAD

INGREDIENTS

2 teaspoons mayonnaise

1 teaspoon chopped fresh chives

¼ teaspoon lemon zest

1 teaspoon lemon juice

1 cup packaged broccoli slaw

Large lettuce leaves

2 hard-boiled large organic cage-free eggs, sliced

2 tablespoons bottled roasted red sweet peppers, drained and
chopped

DIRECTIONS

In a small bowl, combine mayonnaise, chives, lemon zest, and lemon juice. Add broccoli slaw; toss gently to coat. Cover and chill overnight.

Spread broccoli mixture along the bottom edge of a lettuce leaf, leaving 1½ inches on the sides of the leaf. Top with egg slices and roasted red peppers. Season with pepper, if desired.

Fold in the sides of lettuce over the filling. Starting from the bottom edge, roll up.

MAKES 1 SERVING

CLEANSING SPRING SOUP

INGREDIENTS

1 head lettuce, 1 bunch of spinach, or other fresh greens of
   choice
1 carrot, cut into large chunks
1 celery rib, cut into large chunks
1 avocado, cut into chunks
½ tomato, cut into chunks
1 cucumber, peeled and cut into chunks
2–3 scallions, chopped into large pieces
1–2 tablespoons extra-virgin olive oil
1–2 tablespoons umeboshi plum vinegar (or vinegar of
   choice)
1 tablespoon ground cumin
1 tablespoon ground coriander
2–4 cups veggie or chicken broth (or water)
¼ teaspoon cayenne pepper (optional)
½ teaspoon turmeric (optional)
1 clove garlic (optional)
1 cup yogurt or kefir (optional)

DIRECTIONS

Place all ingredients in a blender. It works a little better if you place
the larger items in first, followed by the greens, then pour the liquids and seasonings on top. Blend.

Adjust seasonings. Add salt and pepper, if desired. Blend until
smooth and creamy.

MAKES 4 TO 6 SERVINGS

WILD SALMON SALAD WRAPS

INGREDIENTS

    2–3 tablespoons mayonnaise

    ¼ cup diced celery

    2 tablespoons finely sliced scallions

    4 tablespoons chopped dill

    Zest and juice of ½ lemon

    2 (7.5-ounce) cans wild salmon, drained

    4 medium collard leaves, stem removed at the base of leaf

      (nori wrap or large leaf kale or other green may be used)

DIRECTIONS

In a mixing bowl, combine mayonnaise, celery, scallions, dill, lemon zest, and lemon juice. Fold in salmon. Season with salt and pepper.

Place ¼ of the mixture in the center of a collard leaf. Fold in the sides and roll like a burrito.

MAKES 2 TO 4 SERVINGS

SESAME SEED CHICKEN SALAD

INGREDIENTS

3 organic or pasture-raised boneless, skinless chicken breasts
(about 2 pounds)
Zest and juice of 1 lemon
½ cup mayonnaise
⅓ cup sour cream or Greek yogurt (optional)
1 tablespoon Dijon mustard
1 stalk celery, chopped
½ cup pecans, almonds, or walnuts, chopped and toasted
¼ cup chopped fresh chives
1½ tablespoons sesame seeds
½ cup dried apricots, chopped (optional)

DIRECTIONS

Brine chicken (optional): Make brining liquid by dissolving ¼ cup salt into 1 quart of water. Place chicken breasts in brine for 15 to 30 minutes. Remove from brine and pat dry. Discard brine.

Cover chicken with cold water in a deep skillet or medium-size pot and add 1 teaspoon salt. Bring to a boil over high heat, then reduce the heat to medium-low and simmer, uncovered, until the chicken is cooked through, about 15 minutes. Remove the chicken and let cool.

Place lemon zest and juice into a large bowl. Stir in the mayonnaise, sour cream (if using), mustard, celery, nuts, chives, sesame seeds, ½ teaspoon salt, and pepper to taste. Add the apricots, if using.

Dice the chicken into small pieces and toss with the dressing. Serve with salad.

MAKES 4 SERVINGS

GREEK SALAD

INGREDIENTS

4–5 medium tomatoes, sliced

1 large cucumber, peeled and sliced

1 medium green pepper, deseeded and sliced

1 small red onion, peeled and sliced

4 teaspoons dried oregano

16 olives, ideally Kalamata

4 tablespoons capers (or additional olives)

1 cup crumbled feta cheese (optional)

4 tablespoons extra-virgin olive oil

Fresh oregano leaves (optional)

DIRECTIONS

Place vegetables into a bowl and toss with the dried oregano. Add the olives and capers. Add the feta cheese, if using. Drizzle with oil. Garnish with fresh oregano, if using. Serve on its own or with a protein choice added.

MAKES 4 SERVINGS

TUNA AND MAYONNAISE
STUFFED AVOCADO

INGREDIENTS

4 avocados, halved and pitted
3 (3-ounce cans) tuna, drained
1 tablespoon mayonnaise
1 red bell pepper, diced
1 jalapeño, minced
1 cup cilantro leaves, roughly chopped
Juice of 1 lime

DIRECTIONS

Scoop out some of the avocado from the pitted area to widen the
"bowl" area. Place the scooped avocado into a medium bowl. Mash
it with a fork.

Add the tuna, mayonnaise bell pepper, jalapeño, and cilantro to
the mixing bowl.

Pour lime juice over. Stir it all together until everything is well
mixed. Season with salt and pepper. Scoop the tuna into the avocado bowls.

MAKES 4 SERVINGS

AVOCADO STUFFED WITH CHICKEN SALAD

INGREDIENTS

    1 cup diced cooked organic or pasture-raised chicken breast

    2 tablespoons mayonnaise

    1 teaspoon orange zest

    1 tablespoon chopped shallots

    1 tablespoon chopped red bell pepper

    1 teaspoon chopped fresh chives

    1 avocado, halved and pitted

    4 radicchio leaves

DIRECTIONS

In a bowl combine chicken, mayonnaise, orange zest, shallots, red pepper, and chives. Season to taste with salt and pepper.

Divide the salad between the two avocado halves, filling the cavity.

To serve, place 2 radicchio leaves on each serving plate and top with an avocado half.

MAKES 2 SERVINGS

SALMON SALAD STUFFED AVOCADO

INGREDIENTS

2 small salmon fillets

1 tablespoon organic ghee or coconut oil, melted

2 tablespoons fresh lemon juice

1 small white onion, finely chopped

¼ cup sour cream, crème fraîche, or mayonnaise

1–2 tablespoons chopped fresh dill

1 large or 2 small avocados

Lemon wedges for garnish

DIRECTIONS

Preheat the oven to 400°F. Place the salmon fillets on a baking sheet lined with parchment paper. Drizzle with melted ghee. Season with salt and pepper and 1 tablespoon fresh lemon juice. Place in the oven and bake for 20 to 25 minutes, until cooked through.

Remove the salmon from the oven and let it cool for 5 to 10 minutes. Using a fork, shred the salmon fillets and discard the skin.

Mix the salmon with the onion, sour cream, and dill in a bowl. Add the remaining 1 tablespoon lemon juice, and season with salt and pepper.

Scoop out the middle of the avocado, leaving ½–1 inch of the avocado flesh. Cut the scooped avocado into small pieces.

Place the chopped avocado into the bowl with the salmon and mix until well combined.

Fill each avocado half with the salmon and avocado mixture. Garnish with the lemon wedge.

MAKES 2 SERVINGS

DIY KETO-GREEN SALAD

INGREDIENTS

4 handfuls fresh greens (super greens like kale, parsley, dandelion, spinach, etc.)

4 tomatoes, sliced

1 cucumber, peeled and chopped

Dressing, enough to coat salad (see page 249)

Sprouts (broccoli or other)

Sunflower seeds or slivered almonds

4 pieces salmon, chicken, tuna, or beef; 4 sardines; or 4 hard-boiled eggs, each sliced in half

DIRECTIONS

In a mixing bowl, combine vegetables and toss with dressing. Arrange on 4 plates. Top each with sprouts, sunflower seeds or almonds, and your choice of protein.

MAKES 4 SERVINGS

OTHER OPTIONS FOR DIY KETO-GREEN SALAD

The possibilities are endless for creating delicious salads! This is an easy guideline to make your Keto-Green Salad anytime, any way, as a meal or a side. Get creative and healthy!

Always start with a base that includes dark leafy greens and low-carbohydrate veggies. Good examples are mixed lettuces, arugula, dandelion greens, parsley, kale, spinach, and cabbage.

Top the base with cruciferous vegetables, including broccoli, cauliflower, or cabbage. Add other vegetables of choice, such as watercress, carrots, celery, cucumbers, bell peppers, artichokes, onions, and scallions.

Next comes a layer of 4 to 6 ounces of your choice of protein: shrimp, organic free-range chicken, free-range meat, fish, organic cage-free hard-boiled eggs, non-GMO tempeh, and so forth.

Finally come your healthy fats, including avocado, nuts, and seeds (ground flaxseeds and sesame seeds are tasty choices). You can also top the salad off with sprouts and herbs. Examples include broccoli sprouts, alfalfa sprouts, ginger, oregano, thyme, mint, or cilantro.

For dressing, simply mix together oil and lemon juice with crushed garlic and sea salt.

That's it: your Keto-Green Salad hierarchy.

KETO-GREEN COLESLAW

INGREDIENTS

1 pound green cabbage, shredded

½ medium to large red onion, thinly sliced

1 carrot, grated

1 cup Vegenaise or mayonnaise

¼ cup apple cider vinegar

½ teaspoon ground celery seed

½ teaspoon sea salt

½ teaspoon pepper

Paprika, for garnish

DIRECTIONS

Combine cabbage, onion, and carrot in a large mixing bowl. In a separate bowl, mix together the Vegenaise, vinegar, celery seed, salt, and pepper.

Pour dressing onto vegetables and toss until thoroughly combined. Garnish top with a sprinkle of paprika.

MAKES 4 TO 6 SERVINGS

SALAD DRESSINGS

DR. ANNA'S LEMON GARLIC VINAIGRETTE

INGREDIENTS
1 teaspoon sea salt
3 cloves garlic
2 tablespoons lemon juice
⅔ cup extra-virgin olive oil

DIRECTIONS
The first option is the method I use: With a mortar and pestle, mash the salt and garlic until the garlic is emulsified. Transfer to a bowl, then add the lemon juice and olive oil and stir well. Taste to see if more salt, lemon juice, or EVOO is needed, and adjust accordingly. I've been making this since I was a young girl and it is so yummy and good for you. It makes everything taste better. You can put it on salads, sandwiches, chicken, and fish. Make extra and refrigerate.

The second option is to place all ingredients except the oil in a blender or small food processor and puree until smooth. Pour the mixture into a bowl, then add the olive oil and whisk until emulsified.

BASIL THYME VINAIGRETTE

INGREDIENTS

½ cup balsamic vinegar

2 teaspoons Dijon mustard

3 cloves garlic

¼ cup fresh basil

2 sprigs fresh thyme, leaves removed from stems

⅔ cup extra-virgin olive oil

DIRECTIONS

Place all ingredients except the oil in a blender or small food processor and puree until smooth.

With the blender running, slowly pour in the oil in a steady stream.

Continue blending for 15 seconds to fully incorporate the oil. (Alternatively, you can finely mince the garlic and whisk it together with the other ingredients. Slowly pour in the olive oil, whisking continuously until emulsified.)

SIDE DISHES

ZOODLES (ZUCCHINI NOODLES)

INGREDIENTS

Several whole zucchini

DIRECTIONS

Remove stems from the zucchini. Use a spiralizer to turn the zucchini into noodle-like strips.

Place the zoodles into a steamer and steam lightly until slightly soft. Alternatively, you can sauté them in olive oil until slightly soft.

Season with salt and pepper to taste.

ZOODLES WITH AVOCADO PESTO

INGREDIENTS

1 tablespoon oil or 2 tablespoons organic butter

2 medium zucchini, prepared into zoodles via spiralizer or
thinly sliced

1 avocado

½ cup basil leaves, tightly packed

Juice of ½ lemon or lime

1 clove garlic

¼–⅓ cup extra-virgin olive oil

DIRECTIONS

For zoodles: Heat a large sauté pan over medium heat and add oil
or butter. Add raw zoodles and a little water and cook until tender
but al dente, stirring occasionally with tongs. (Or you can use a
steamer to cook the zoodles.)

For avocado pesto: Place the avocado, basil, lemon juice, and
garlic in a food processor or blender and blend until smooth. With
the motor running, slowly add the oil.

In a large bowl, thoroughly combine zoodles with the sauce.
Delicious! You may never want pasta again!

MAKES 2 TO 4 SERVINGS

CAULIFLOWER MASH

INGREDIENTS

> 1 to 2 heads organic cauliflower (depending on size), stems removed and florets separated
> 3 to 4 tablespoons organic butter or ghee
> ½ teaspoon sea salt

DIRECTIONS

Boil the cauliflower with the salt. When soft, drain, add butter, and mash well. Add more butter, if desired. Salt and pepper to taste. You will love this more than mashed potatoes from now on and feel even better after eating it!

MAKES 4 SERVINGS

SCENTED CAULIFLOWER RICE

INGREDIENTS

1 head organic cauliflower, stem removed

2 tablespoons organic butter or coconut oil

1 tablespoon cumin seeds

1 cup diced onion

2 cloves garlic, minced

1 teaspoon sea salt

1 teaspoon black pepper

Zest and juice of 2 limes

DIRECTIONS

Rinse cauliflower under cool water and pat dry.

Break the cauliflower into florets, removing the stems. Place the florets in a food processor bowl and pulse until the cauliflower looks like rice. This takes about 10 to 15 pulses. You may need to do this in two batches.

Heat the butter or coconut oil in a skillet over medium heat.

Add the cumin seeds and sauté for 1 minute.

Add the onion and garlic and cook, stirring occasionally, for 3 to 4 minutes, or until the onion is relatively translucent.

Add cauliflower rice and continue to sauté for 4 to 5 minutes.

Remove from heat. Add salt, pepper, and lime zest and juice, and mix well.

MAKES 4 SERVINGS

MEXI-CAULI RICE

INGREDIENTS

1 head organic cauliflower, stem removed

2 tablespoons organic butter or coconut oil

1 teaspoon cumin seeds or powder

1 teaspoon chili powder

2 cloves garlic, minced

1 tomato, diced

DIRECTIONS

Rinse cauliflower under cool water and pat dry.

Break the cauliflower into florets, removing the stems. Place the florets in a food processor bowl and pulse until the cauliflower looks like rice. This takes about 10 to 15 pulses. You may need to do this in two batches.

Heat the butter or coconut oil in a skillet over medium heat.

Add the cumin seeds and sauté for 1 minute.

Add the chili powder, garlic, and tomato and cook, stirring occasionally, 2 to 3 minutes.

Add cauliflower rice and continue to sauté for 4 to 5 minutes.

Season with salt and pepper. Remove from heat and serve.

MAKES 4 SERVINGS

SAUTÉED GREENS

INGREDIENTS

1 bunch greens (arugula, Swiss chard, kale, collard greens, mustard greens, dandelion greens, spinach, or any other)

2 tablespoons organic butter

1–2 tablespoons extra-virgin olive oil, divided

1–2 tablespoons lemon juice and/or apple cider vinegar

DIRECTIONS

Wash and dry greens. If using greens with large leaves, place three or more leaves on top of each other, roll, and slice into 1-inch strips, then slice once more lengthwise. Continue until all greens are cut.

Heat butter in a large skillet over medium heat.

Add greens to skillet. You may have to add in batches. Toss with half of the oil and cook until wilted and tender, about 4 to 5 minutes.

Remove from skillet and place in bowl. Toss with the rest of the olive oil and the lemon juice and/or vinegar. Season with salt and pepper.

MAKES 4 SERVINGS

SAUTÉED BEET GREENS

INGREDIENTS

2 cups or more beet greens (beet greens are my favorite, as they really alkalinize me)

1 tablespoon organic butter or ghee

2 cloves garlic, chopped

½ onion, very thinly sliced

½ cup extra-virgin olive oil

1 teaspoon sea salt

Cayenne pepper or sriracha sauce (optional)

Juice of 1 lemon (removes the bitterness from the greens)

DIRECTIONS

Wash beet greens thoroughly. Cut greens into 4-inch segments, along with stems.

Heat ghee in a skillet over medium heat. Add garlic and onion and sauté until tender. Add beet greens and cook for 20 minutes, uncovered.

Place in serving dish, drizzle with olive oil, add salt, and mix well. Add cayenne pepper or sriracha, if using. Squeeze lemon juice over the greens.

MAKES 1 TO 2 SERVINGS

ROASTED SPRING VEGGIES

INGREDIENTS

1 pound assorted spring vegetables (such as carrots, asparagus, radishes, baby summer squashes, spring onions, or
sugar snap peas), trimmed or peeled or cut into bite-sized
pieces

4 garlic cloves, minced

2 tablespoons extra-virgin olive oil

DIRECTIONS

Preheat the oven to 450°F.

Line a rimmed baking sheet with parchment paper.

Combine vegetables, garlic, and oil in a large bowl. Season with
salt and pepper; toss to coat.

Spread the veggies out in a single layer on a baking sheet. Roast
for 20 minutes, stir, then roast an additional 10 to 15 minutes until
tender, golden brown, and charred in spots.

Serve warm or at room temperature.

MAKES 4 TO 6 SERVINGS

EASY KETO-GREEN VEGGIE SAUTÉ

Here's an easy way to build a simple veggie dish and quick and delicious Keto-Green meal:

Add oil, organic ghee or butter, or bacon first to a saucepan, and heat.

For your next layer, add onions, leeks, garlic, or shallots—all of which help your liver detoxify.

Next, sprinkle in spices, including sea salt and pepper, turmeric, cumin or allspice, garam masala, coriander or ginger. You choose your favorites.

Then layer in the vegetables you prefer, starting with the ones with the longest cooking times. An approximate order would be: cabbage, Brussels sprouts, and carrots, followed by eggplant and mushrooms. Last to go in would be cauliflower, daikon radishes, broccoli, zucchini, yellow squash, bell pepper, bok choy, celery, bamboo shoots, and artichokes, in that order. Cook each layer for a few minutes, until partially tender, before adding the next layer.

Add a layer of greens. Cook until the greens are soft but still have a vibrant color.

As an option, add 1 tablespoon apple cider vinegar and additional seasoning to taste.

Voilà—you have created a tasty, amazing Keto-Green vegetable dish. Now you can top it with your protein of choice for a complete meal. Often I will remove the veggies and cook the protein in the same pan to pick up the flavors (and have less to clean up!).

CRUCIFEROUS VEGGIE BAKE

INGREDIENTS

    1 cup chopped kale
    1 cup broccoli florets
    1 cup Brussels sprouts, halved
    1 cup chopped red cabbage
    1 stick organic butter, melted
    3 cloves garlic, mashed
    ½–1 teaspoon sea salt
    1 teaspoon allspice
    ¼ cup pine nuts or slivered almonds (optional)

DIRECTIONS

    Preheat the oven to 375°F.

    In a glass baking dish, combine the vegetables.

    In a separate bowl, blend the butter with garlic, sea salt, and allspice. Pour butter mixture over veggies and combine well.

    Add pine nuts or slivered almonds to the mixture of veggies.

    Bake for 45 minutes or until all veggies are soft. Eat hot or cold.

    Optional: Add a protein of choice to serve alongside.

MAKES 4 TO 6 SERVINGS

BROCCOLI WITH LEMON SAUCE

INGREDIENTS

    4 cups broccoli, sliced

    1 tablespoon organic butter

    1 tablespoon extra-virgin olive oil

    1 teaspoon Italian-style seasoning

    Zest and juice of ½ lemon

    ¼ teaspoon salt

DIRECTIONS

Steam the broccoli for 3 to 5 minutes, until tender but still al dente.

Meanwhile, in a small saucepan over medium-low heat, combine the butter, oil, Italian seasoning, lemon zest and juice, and salt. Cook for 2 minutes.

Place the broccoli in a bowl and toss with the lemon sauce before serving.

MAKES 4 SERVINGS

BACON-WRAPPED ASPARAGUS

INGREDIENTS

1 bunch asparagus

1 pound bacon

DIRECTIONS

Preheat the oven to 350°F. Line a rimmed baking sheet with parchment paper.

Wash asparagus and cut or snap off stem approximately 1 inch from the end. Wrap asparagus (3 if thin, or 1–2 if thick) with 1 strip bacon. Place on baking sheet. Bake 15 minutes; then flip them over. Turn oven to broil and broil for 3 to 5 minutes.

MAKES 4 SERVINGS

MAIN DISHES

KETO-GREEN CROCK-POT
LAMB AND VEGGIE STEW

INGREDIENTS

Boneless lamb leg roast (3–4 pounds)

1 tablespoon organic ghee

½ cup chicken broth

6 cloves garlic, minced

2–3 sprigs rosemary, leaves only, chopped

2–3 sprigs thyme, leaves only, chopped

⅓ cup stone-ground mustard

2 carrots, peeled and chopped

2 cups whole white mushrooms

2 stalks celery, cut in 1-inch pieces

2 large onions, peeled and quartered

(You may choose to add other veggies as well, since we've omitted potatoes and other starchy vegetables. Some good choices are: cauliflower and broccoli—including the stalks—swiss chard with stems, cabbage, and bok choy.)

DIRECTIONS

Dry the lamb very well with paper towels. Season generously with salt and pepper. Heat a cast-iron skillet over high heat, then add the ghee. Sear the meat for 3 to 4 minutes on each side. Remove the meat from the pan. Reduce the heat to medium, and add the chicken broth, scraping up the brown bits from the bottom of the pan. Turn off and set aside.

Place the roast in a slow cooker.

In a small bowl, mix the garlic, rosemary, thyme, and mustard. Pour it over the lamb and use your hands to coat the meat with the mixture.

Toss the carrots, mushrooms, celery, and onions with salt and pepper, and arrange them around the meat. Pour the chicken broth from the pan on top of the veggies.

Cook on low for 8 to 10 hours.

Option: I love to cook in my pressure cooker. It saves time and creates really tender meat. Do what works best for you. You could also make this recipe on the stove top or in the oven.

Serve with a green salad or side of asparagus.

MAKES 4 TO 6 SERVINGS

SPICY CHICKEN (OR TEMPEH) STIR-FRY

INGREDIENTS

1 pound chicken, cubed (or organic tempeh, sliced)

1 teaspoon red curry sauce

1 teaspoon paprika

1 tablespoon grated fresh ginger

4 garlic cloves, minced

2 tablespoons plus 1 teaspoon low-sodium soy sauce
   or tamari

2 tablespoons rice vinegar

2 tablespoons toasted sesame oil

2 tablespoons avocado oil

1 medium red onion, slivered

2 cups cauliflower florets, cut into smaller pieces

1 yellow bell pepper, cut into strips

1 cup snow peas

¼ cup low-sodium vegetable broth (or water)

1 teaspoon red pepper flakes

1 tablespoon sesame seeds, for garnish

DIRECTIONS

Combine the chicken (or sliced tempeh) with the red curry sauce, paprika, ginger, garlic, 2 tablespoons of the tamari, vinegar, and sesame oil in a glass bowl. Marinate in the refrigerator for at least 30 minutes and up to 12 hours.

Preheat the oven to 350°F.

Place the marinated chicken (or tempeh) on a parchment-lined rimmed baking sheet. Drizzle the remaining marinade on top. Bake for 30 minutes.

After 30 minutes, remove the baking sheet from the oven (the marinade should have dried but not burned).

Meanwhile, heat a sauté pan over medium-high heat. Add the avocado oil and onion and sauté, stirring occasionally, for 2 minutes, until the onion softens. Add the cauliflower and sauté for another 2 minutes. Add the bell pepper, snow peas, remaining 1 teaspoon tamari, vegetable broth, and red pepper flakes.

Reduce the heat to medium, cover the pan, and simmer for another 4 to 5 minutes, until the vegetables are tender.

Remove from the heat and garnish with the sesame seeds.

MAKES 4 SERVINGS

BEEF KEBOBS

INGREDIENTS

    1 pound grass-fed steak, cubed

    1–2 green, red, or yellow bell peppers, cut in chunks

    1–2 tomatoes, cut in chunks

    1 cup whole mushrooms

    1 onion, cut in chunks

    Onion salt

DIRECTIONS

Marinate or season the steak to your liking, if desired. Place cubes on skewers, alternating with the vegetables. Sprinkle with onion salt.

    Grill to desired doneness. Serve with a side of fresh greens.

MAKES 4 SERVINGS

STIR-FRY SHRIMP WITH EGGPLANT AND ONIONS

INGREDIENTS

2 tablespoons minced fresh ginger

2 garlic cloves, minced

½ tablespoon coconut oil

¼ cup vegetable broth

½ teaspoon sesame oil

1 tablespoon mirin (optional)

3 tablespoons low-sodium soy sauce or tamari

Crushed red pepper (optional)

¾ pound frozen shrimp, defrosted, peeled, and deveined

2 tablespoons grapeseed oil or organic butter, divided

1 carrot, peeled and sliced diagonally

1 medium onion, chopped

1 green pepper, chopped

1 large eggplant, chopped

2 green onions, sliced diagonally

DIRECTIONS

Combine ginger, garlic, and coconut oil in a small bowl. Set aside.

Whisk together the vegetable broth, sesame oil, mirin, soy sauce, and crushed red pepper if using. Set sauce aside.

Pat shrimp dry with a paper towel. Season with salt and pepper.

Heat a wok over medium-high heat and add 1 tablespoon of the grapeseed oil (or butter). Add shrimp. Cook without turning, 1 to 2 minutes. Turn shrimp and cook 3 to 5 minutes more, until done. Remove shrimp and set aside.

Add ¼ cup water to the wok and add carrots. Cover and cook for 2 minutes. Remove carrots and add to the plate with the shrimp. Discard any excess water and wipe the wok clean with a paper towel.

Turn heat down to medium and add remaining 1 tablespoon grapeseed oil (or butter) to the wok. Add onions, peppers, and eggplant and cook for 4 to 6 minutes. Move vegetables to the edges of the wok. Add ginger-garlic mixture to the middle of the wok and cook 90 seconds. Combine ginger-garlic mixture with the vegetables in the wok.

Add sauce and mix into vegetables thoroughly. Cook 1 to 2 minutes, until the sauce is reduced. Add shrimp and carrots back to the wok, toss to coat, and cook for another 1 to 2 minutes, until heated through. Garnish with green onions and serve over cooked cauliflower rice.

MAKES 4 SERVINGS

CARDAMOM SEARED SCALLOPS WITH ZOODLES AND AVOCADO PESTO

INGREDIENTS

1 avocado, cut into chunks

½ cup basil leaves, tightly packed

Juice of ½ lemon or lime

1 garlic clove

¼ cup extra-virgin olive oil

2 medium zucchini, prepared (spiralized) into zoodles

4–6 ounces large sea scallops, muscle removed and patted dry

2 tablespoons ground cardamom

1 tablespoon extra-virgin olive oil

DIRECTIONS

To make sauce, combine avocado, basil, lemon juice, and garlic clove in a food processor or blender and blend into a paste. With the motor running, slowly add ¼ cup oil and blend until smooth.

Place raw zoodles in a large sauté pan with a little water and cook until tender but al dente, stirring occasionally with tongs. (You can also use a steamer to cook the zoodles.)

Coat scallops evenly on both sides with cardamom, and season with salt and pepper.

In a large sauté pan, heat oil on medium-high to high heat. Sear the scallops on one side, without moving, until a golden crust forms, about 2 to 3 minutes. Turn scallops and sear on the other side.

In a mixing bowl, combine zoodles with sauce and divide among 4 plates. Top each portion of zoodles with a portion of scallops.

MAKES 4 SERVINGS

GRILLED SALMON WITH GARLIC OREGANO AIOLI

INGREDIENTS

2 cloves minced garlic

4 tablespoons extra-virgin olive oil

1 teaspoon minced rosemary

1 teaspoon salt

4 (5-ounce) salmon fillets

Garlic Oregano Aioli (recipe follows)

DIRECTIONS

Preheat the oven to 400°F or heat a grill to high heat.

Combine garlic, oil, rosemary, and salt. Rub salmon with herb–olive oil mixture. Fillets can be marinated in the refrigerator for up to 4 hours.

Place fish on parchment-lined baking sheet for the oven. For grilling, use a cedar plank or grill grid or basket.

Cook for about 8 to 14 minutes, until fish is firm but still tender when poked in the middle.

Serve with Garlic Oregano Aioli.

MAKES 4 SERVINGS

GARLIC OREGANO AIOLI

INGREDIENTS

1 cup mayonnaise

1 tablespoon extra-virgin olive oil

2 teaspoons chopped fresh oregano (marjoram is good too)

2 garlic cloves, pressed or minced

Zest and juice of 1 lemon

DIRECTIONS

Whisk or blend mayonnaise, oil, oregano, garlic, lemon zest and juice in small bowl. Season with salt and pepper. Adjust garlic or lemon if needed.

Cover and chill. Can be made 2 days ahead.

CROCK-POT CHICKEN SOUP

INGREDIENTS

1 whole organic or pasture-raised chicken

2 tablespoons organic butter

1 teaspoon garlic powder

1 teaspoon salt

½ teaspoon each dried basil, oregano, rosemary, and thyme

1 small yellow onion, chopped

1 stalk celery, chopped

1 carrot, chopped

DIRECTIONS

Place chicken in a slow cooker with butter, garlic powder, salt, and herbs. Cook on low for 6 to 8 hours or overnight.

Remove chicken to a plate. When cool enough to handle, remove meat from the bones. Set the meat aside to cool completely, then cover and refrigerate.

Put the bones back in the slow cooker. Add the vegetables and 2 to 3 quarts water. Cook on low for 6 to 8 hours or overnight.

Strain bones and vegetables out of broth. Add chicken meat and reheat.

Store leftovers in the refrigerator for up to 3 days, or freeze for later use.

MAKES 4 TO 6 SERVINGS

CRISPY HERB-ROASTED CHICKEN THIGHS

INGREDIENTS

4 bone-in, skin-on organic or pasture-raised chicken thighs
(or breasts)

4 tablespoons organic butter, softened

¼ cup minced fresh herbs (rosemary and thyme are delicious)

2 cloves garlic, minced

½ teaspoon salt

DIRECTIONS

Preheat the oven to 450°F.

Rinse chicken and pat dry. Place on parchment-lined rimmed baking sheet.

Combine softened butter, half of minced herbs, garlic, and salt.

Rub approximately 1 tablespoon herb butter underneath the skin of each chicken part. Drizzle the chicken with a little olive oil and rub over the skin. Sprinkle with remaining herbs. Season with salt and pepper.

Place in oven and bake for 15 minutes. Reduce heat to 375°F and bake an additional 30 minutes, until an instant-read thermometer reads 180°F or the juices run clear.

MAKES 2 TO 4 SERVINGS

CROCK-POT ROAST BEEF

INGREDIENTS

1 beef roast, 1½ pounds

1 teaspoon black pepper

2 cloves garlic, mashed

⅓ cup tamari

¼ cup balsamic vinegar

2 tablespoons dry mustard

DIRECTIONS

Rub roast with pepper and garlic.

Place in slow cooker with tamari, vinegar, and dry mustard. Cook on slow for 8 hours or on high for 4 hours.

MAKES 4 TO 6 SERVINGS

CORIANDER-CRUSTED RIB EYE STEAKS

INGREDIENTS

2 rib eye steaks, 6 to 8 ounces each

Ground coriander

Salt

Pepper

1 tablespoon organic butter or ghee

DIRECTIONS

Cover each side of the steaks with a generous coating of coriander, salt, and pepper.

Heat a cast-iron skillet over medium-high heat and add butter or ghee.

Cook steaks for about 3 minutes on each side, allowing a nice crust to form on each side. Remove from pan and let rest 5 minutes before carving.

Serve with a side of cruciferous vegetables or cauliflower mash and side salad.

MAKES 2 SERVINGS

FLANK STEAK WITH CHIMICHURRI SAUCE

INGREDIENTS

½ cup extra-virgin olive oil

¼ cup red wine vinegar

2 tablespoons lemon juice

1 cup chopped flat-leaf parsley

4 tablespoons chopped fresh basil

1 tablespoon chopped fresh oregano

2 tablespoons minced garlic

2½ tablespoons minced shallot

1 teaspoon crushed red pepper

1½–2 pounds flank, skirt, or flap steak

DIRECTIONS

To make the sauce, combine in the bowl of a food processor the olive oil, vinegar, lemon juice, parsley, basil, oregano, garlic, and shallots. Pulse until well blended, but without pureeing. Add ½ teaspoon salt, ¼ teaspoon pepper, and the crushed red pepper. Set aside 1 cup sauce and cover with plastic wrap; reserve at room temperature for up to 6 hours.

Season the steak with 1 teaspoon salt and ¼ teaspoon pepper per side and place in a large resealable plastic bag. Add the remaining chimichurri sauce. Seal bag and refrigerate the steak for at least 2 hours.

Preheat a grill to medium heat or heat a cast-iron skillet or grill pan to medium.

Remove the steak from the refrigerator and let it come to room temperature for 30 minutes. Brush the excess chimichurri sauce off the steak and set the steak over the hot grill. Cook 2 to 3 minutes per side, or until desired doneness.

Allow the steak to rest for 5 to 7 minutes before slicing across the grain into 2-inch-wide strips.

Serve with reserved chimichurri sauce and a side of cruciferous vegetables or cauliflower mash and side salad.

MAKES 4 TO 6 SERVINGS

ROSEMARY SEARED LAMB CHOPS

INGREDIENTS

12 lamb loin chops

2 tablespoons minced fresh rosemary

1 tablespoon salt

1 teaspoon pepper

1 tablespoon organic butter or ghee

DIRECTIONS

About an hour before cooking, remove chops from refrigerator to bring to room temperature.

Combine rosemary, salt, and pepper in a small mixing bowl. Cover both sides of the chops with a generous coating of the herb mixture.

Heat a cast-iron skillet over medium-high heat and add butter. Let it get very hot, but not smoking, before adding chops.

Cook chops for about 2 minutes on each side for medium rare or 3 to 4 minutes on each side for more well done, allowing a nice crust to form on each side.

Remove from pan and let rest 5 minutes before serving. Pour pan juices over chops, if desired.

Serve with a side of asparagus or cauliflower mash and side salad.

MAKES 4 SERVINGS

SALMON CAKES

INGREDIENTS

¼ cup white wine

1 teaspoon dill

8 ounces salmon, fresh or canned

1 egg, beaten

2 stalks celery, minced

1 onion, minced

½ bunch cilantro, minced

1 tablespoon minced parsley

½ cup mayonnaise

1 teaspoon ground coriander

1 tablespoon fresh lemon juice

1 cup gluten-free bread crumbs

1 teaspoon sea salt

½ teaspoon white pepper

4 tablespoons organic butter, ghee, or coconut oil

DIRECTIONS

If using fresh salmon, poach fish. Heat wine, ½ cup water, and dill in a sauté pan and bring to a simmer. Place salmon fillets skin-side down in the pan. Cover and cook 5 to 10 minutes, or until fish flakes apart easily. Do not overcook. Remove from pan and let cool. Flake salmon into large chunks and place in a medium-size mixing bowl.

If using canned salmon, drain and flake salmon and place in a medium-size mixing bowl.

Gently combine the fish with the egg, celery, onion, cilantro, parsley, mayonnaise, coriander, lemon juice, ½ cup bread crumbs, salt, and pepper until mixture just clings together.

Divide mixture into 8 portions and shape into flat cakes. Arrange on baking sheet lined with parchment paper; cover with plastic wrap and chill at least 30 minutes. (Can be refrigerated up to 24 hours.)

Put remaining bread crumbs on plate and lightly dredge cakes.

Heat the butter or oil in a skillet over medium-high heat. Gently lay fish cakes in skillet and pan-fry until outsides are crisp and browned, 3 to 4 minutes per side.

MAKES 4 SERVINGS

PAN-ROASTED SALMON

INGREDIENTS

　　1 tablespoon organic ghee or coconut oil
　　1 (5–6-ounce) salmon fillet
　　Lemon juice
　　Dried herbs of choice

DIRECTIONS

　　Heat a frying pan over medium-high heat and add ghee.

　　Season the salmon with salt and pepper. Squeeze a little lemon juice over the fish. Season with the herbs.

　　Cook the fish for 2 to 3 minutes, then turn and cook 1 to 2 minutes more, or until cooked through.

　　Serve with a side of Keto-Green Salad.

MAKES 1 SERVING

PISTACHIO WHITE FISH

INGREDIENTS

2 cloves garlic

1 teaspoon dried oregano

1 teaspoon pepper

½ teaspoon salt

1 to 1½ cups chopped cilantro

⅓ cup pistachios

¼ cup extra-virgin olive oil

1 (6–8-ounce) fillet tilapia, sea bass, or other white fish

2 sheets of natural parchment paper

DIRECTIONS

Preheat the oven to 350°F.

Combine garlic, oregano, pepper, salt, cilantro, and pistachios in a food processor or blender. Blend into a rough paste. With the motor running, add olive oil slowly and blend into a thick paste.

Spread the mixture on the fish. Lay the fish on parchment paper. Cover with another sheet of the paper.

Bake about 18 minutes, until fish flakes easily with a fork.

MAKES 1 SERVING

EASY KETO FRITTATA WITH SAUTÉED SPINACH

INGREDIENTS

20 small asparagus spears

2 tablespoons organic ghee

2 small scallions, chopped

1 small shallot, chopped

1 large red bell pepper, sliced into strips

10 large organic cage-free eggs

¼ cup full-fat whipping cream or coconut whipped cream
(both optional)

2 tablespoons chopped fresh parsley (or 1 teaspoon dried)

2 tablespoons chopped fresh mint (or 1 teaspoon dried)

1 tablespoon chopped fresh tarragon (or 1 teaspoon dried)

1 (4-ounce) package goat cheese (or any soft full-fat cheese)
(optional)

1 (3-ounce) package of pancetta or 8 to 10 slices
of bacon

4 cherry tomatoes, halved

DIRECTIONS

Preheat the oven to 400°F.

Prepare the asparagus by cutting the woody ends off.

Heat a nonstick pan over medium heat and add 1 tablespoon ghee. Add the asparagus, scallions, shallot, and bell pepper. Season with salt. Cook about 5 minutes, then set aside.

In a bowl, whisk the eggs, cream (if using), and herbs. Season with salt and pepper.

Place the cooked vegetables into a baking dish. Crumble the cheese (if using) equally all over the vegetables and pour the egg mixture over them. Place it in the oven and cook about 20 minutes, until the top just becomes firm. Remove the dish from the oven and reduce the temperature to 350°F.

Lay the pancetta or bacon all over the frittata and place back in the oven for an additional 15 to 20 minutes.

Serve with a side of tomatoes drizzled with EVOO and a small amount of balsamic vinegar.

MAKES 4 SERVINGS

CHICKEN WINGS WITH BUFFALO SAUCE

INGREDIENTS

24 organic or pasture-raised chicken wings

1 tablespoon aluminum-free baking powder

½ teaspoon salt

¼ teaspoon pepper

¼ cup extra-virgin olive oil

½ cup tomato sauce

6 medium garlic cloves, minced

1 teaspoon Italian-style seasoning

1 teaspoon paprika

Cayenne pepper

DIRECTIONS

Preheat the oven to 400°F.

In a bowl, combine the chicken with the baking powder. Season with the salt and pepper. Place the wings on a roasting tray and bake for 35 to 40 minutes, until the chicken is browned. Remove the chicken and reduce oven temperature to 350°F.

Meanwhile, combine the oil, tomato sauce, garlic, Italian seasoning, paprika, and cayenne to taste in a separate large bowl.

Stir the browned chicken in the bowl of sauce until the wings are well coated.

Return to the roasting tray and bake for another 12 minutes.

Serve with a side of coleslaw, kimchi, or sauerkraut.

MAKES 4 SERVINGS

OVEN-ROASTED RATATOUILLE

INGREDIENTS

1 medium-large red onion, cut into 8 wedges

1 large eggplant, peeled and cut into 1-inch chunks

1 medium-large zucchini, cut into 1-inch chunks

1 medium-large yellow squash, cut into 1-inch chunks

4 plum tomatoes, quartered

8 ounces crimini mushrooms, quartered

1 red bell pepper, seeds removed, cut into 1-inch chunks

4 cloves garlic, chopped

¼ cup Kalamata olives, pitted

½ cup canned or jarred artichoke hearts, quartered

2 tablespoons extra-virgin olive oil

1 tablespoon fresh thyme (or 1 teaspoon dried)

½ tablespoon fresh rosemary (or ½ teaspoon dried)

¼ cup roughly chopped flat-leaf parsley

DIRECTIONS

Preheat the oven to 400°F.

Toss everything together in a large mixing bowl except the parsley. Evenly coat the vegetables with the oil and seasonings.

Roast the coated vegetables in the oven on a rimmed baking sheet for 35 to 40 minutes, or until vegetables are very tender. Toss with parsley.

Serve with sliced avocado and/or top with an over-easy fried egg, if desired.

MAKES 4 SERVINGS

TURKEY TENDERS WITH
MIDDLE EASTERN SPICES

INGREDIENTS

    1 pound organic, cage-free turkey tenders, sliced into
      1-inch-thick strips (you could alternatively make this recipe
      with beef strips, chicken, fish, or tempeh too—it's a favor-
      ite!)

    2 tablespoons avocado oil

    2 tablespoons fresh lemon juice

    ¼ teaspoon ground cardamom

    ½ teaspoon ground cumin

    ½ teaspoon ground turmeric

    ¼ teaspoon ground cinnamon

    2 garlic cloves, minced

    ¼ cup chopped fresh mint

DIRECTIONS

Combine the turkey strips with 1 tablespoon oil, the lemon juice,
spices, garlic, and all but 1 tablespoon of the mint. Season with salt
and pepper and marinate, covered, for 20 to 60 minutes.

Heat a sauté pan over medium-high heat. Add the remaining
1 tablespoon oil, then the turkey, and sauté, turning occasionally,
until cooked through. Remove the turkey from the pan and garnish with the remaining mint.

Serve with your Keto-Green side dish of choice.

MAKES 4 SERVINGS

CHICKEN OR TURKEY CHILI

INGREDIENTS

16-ounce (1 package) ground free-range chicken or turkey

4 cups chicken broth

2 cloves garlic, minced

1 medium yellow onion, diced

2 medium poblano peppers, diced

1 (4-ounce) can diced green chiles, with liquid

1 teaspoon ground cumin

½ teaspoon ground coriander

½ teaspoon chili powder

½ teaspoon dried oregano

1 teaspoon salt

1 teaspoon freshly ground black pepper

Lime wedges, for serving

½ cup coarsely chopped cilantro, for serving

DIRECTIONS

Combine all ingredients except lime wedges and cilantro in a 4- to 6-quart slow cooker. Cook on low for 8 hours or on high for 4 hours.

Mix well.

Garnish with lime wedges and cilantro.

Serve with cauliflower rice, if desired.

Save leftovers, as this is always better the second day!

MAKES 4 SERVINGS

NUT AND SEED NO-MEAT BALLS WITH ZUCCHINI NOODLES

INGREDIENTS

   2 tablespoons extra-virgin olive oil

   1 medium yellow onion, diced

   ½ cup diced celery

   2 cloves garlic, chopped

   ½ pound mushrooms, coarsely chopped

   1 tablespoon each almonds, walnuts, and sunflower seeds,
      very finely chopped

   1 tablespoon extra-virgin olive oil

   1 tablespoon nutritional yeast

   1 tablespoon ground flaxseeds

   1 teaspoon each dried oregano, thyme, and sage

   2 tablespoons almond flour

   2 medium zucchini, spiralized into zoodles (see recipe on page 254)

DIRECTIONS

Preheat the oven to 350°F. Line 2 large baking sheets with parchment paper.

Heat a large sauté pan over medium heat. Add 2 tablespoons oil and onions, celery, and garlic. Sauté 2 to 3 minutes until they begin to soften. Add mushrooms and sauté 4 to 5 minutes, stirring occasionally. Remove from heat and set aside.

Meanwhile, in a food processor, add all remaining ingredients through almond flour and pulse until coarsely ground; be careful not to overprocess. Place into a mixing bowl.

Add the sautéed veggies to the nut mixture and mix by hand until incorporated. Set the mixture aside for 5 to 10 minutes.

Using your hands, form 1-inch balls and place them on the baking sheets.

Bake for 30 minutes until crispy on the outside and soft in the middle. Serve with zoodles and Italian Tomato Sauce.

MAKES 2 SERVINGS

ITALIAN TOMATO SAUCE

INGREDIENTS

Small yellow onion, diced

2 garlic cloves, minced

1 (28-ounce) can crushed tomatoes

2 tablespoons fresh chopped basil (or 1 teaspoon dried)

1 teaspoon dried oregano

1 teaspoon liquid coconut aminos

DIRECTIONS

Heat a saucepan over medium heat and add olive oil. Sauté the onion and garlic 4 to 5 minutes, until softened. Add tomatoes, basil, oregano, and coconut aminos. Simmer for 15 minutes. Season with salt and pepper.

MAKES 4 SERVINGS

TURKEY MEATBALLS IN
EASY TOMATO SAUCE

INGREDIENTS

    1 pound ground free-range turkey
    1 small yellow onion, chopped
    ½ cup chopped parsley
    1 large, organic, free-range egg
    1 teaspoon dried oregano

DIRECTIONS

Preheat the oven to 350°F.

Mix all ingredients together, and shape into golf-ball-size meatballs. Bake in the oven for 25 minutes, until cooked through.

EASY TOMATO SAUCE

INGREDIENTS

    4 cloves garlic, minced
    4 large tomatoes, chopped
    Italian-style seasoning, to taste

DIRECTIONS

Sauté garlic in olive oil until golden, being careful not to burn it. Add tomatoes and seasoning to taste. Bring to a boil. Lower heat and simmer for 15 minutes.

Add the baked meatballs to the sauce.

MAKES 4 SERVINGS

LETTUCE TACOS

INGREDIENTS

½ pound free-range ground beef

1 small yellow onion, chopped

1 tablespoon coconut oil

2 teaspoons chili powder

1 teaspoon salt

Romaine lettuce leaves

1 avocado, sliced

1 handful cilantro, chopped

1 tomato, chopped

Sour cream (optional)

DIRECTIONS

Sauté the ground beef with onion, coconut oil, chili powder, and salt until browned.

Place mixture in lettuce leaves and top with avocado, cilantro, and tomato. Roll up like a burrito. Top with sour cream, if using.

MAKES 2 TO 4 SERVINGS

OVEN-BRAISED SPARE RIBS

INGREDIENTS

   1 tablespoon smoked paprika

   1 tablespoon dried thyme

   ½ tablespoon ground cumin

   1 teaspoon salt

   ½ tablespoon cracked black pepper

   2 pounds spare ribs, cut into 4 pieces

   2 tablespoons organic ghee or oil (not coconut oil)

   Small yellow onion, sliced

   2 cloves garlic, minced

   1 (4-ounce) can tomato paste

   2 tablespoons apple cider vinegar

   4 cups beef stock or bone broth

DIRECTIONS

Preheat the oven to 375°F.

In a small bowl, combine paprika, thyme, cumin, salt, and pepper. Coat ribs evenly on both sides with spice mixture.

In a large oven-safe Dutch oven or braising pan, heat ghee over medium-high heat. Place ribs meaty side down and cook 3 to 4 minutes, until browned. Turn and brown other side. Remove ribs from pan and set aside.

Add onions and garlic to pan and cook until translucent. Add tomato paste, vinegar, and broth and whisk until blended. Return ribs to pan and coat with sauce. Cover pan and bake for 2½ hours.

Serve with Keto-Green side dish of choice. I suggest cauliflower mash and a side salad.

MAKES 4 SERVINGS

DRINKS

KETO COFFEE OR TEA

INGREDIENTS
1 cup brewed coffee or tea
1 tablespoon coconut oil or MCT oil
1 teaspoon unsalted organic ghee

OPTIONAL ADDITIONS
1 egg yolk
1 teaspoon to 1 tablespoon hydrolyzed gelatin or powdered
  collagen (which does not cause liquids to gel)
¼ teaspoon cinnamon and/or cardamom
1–5 drops of stevia, monkfruit-based sweetener, or pure
  vanilla extract

DIRECTIONS

Place all ingredients in a blender; pulse until smooth. Pour into a mug and enjoy.

MAKES 1 SERVING

Note: If you're concerned about the potential risk of salmonella in raw egg yolks, you can make them safe by using pasteurized eggs. To pasteurize eggs at home, simply pour enough water in a saucepan to cover the eggs. Heat the water to 140°F. Using a spoon, slowly lower the eggs into the water. Keep the eggs in the water for about 3 minutes. This should be enough to pasteurize the eggs and kill any potential bacteria without cooking the eggs. Remove the eggs from the water, let cool, and store in the fridge for 6 to 8 weeks.

DR. ANNA'S TE-KETO COCKTAIL

Tequila and potato vodka have quite a low glycemic index, so they can be enjoyed in the occasional refreshing cocktail without it being likely to kick you out of ketosis. Sometimes I add a zing by muddling in a fresh jalapeño slice and fresh ginger.

INGREDIENTS

1–2 ounces tequila

Juice of ½ lime

DIRECTIONS

Pour the tequila into a shaker cup with ice. Squeeze lime into the tequila. Shake hard. Strain and serve up in a salt-rimmed glass or on ice.

MAKES 1 SERVING

DR. ANNA'S KOOL KETO MOCKTAIL

INGREDIENTS

Fresh mint

Lime or lemon, cut in wedges

Ice

Sparkling water

Pomegranate seeds (optional)

DIRECTIONS

In a large glass, muddle together mint and lime or lemon. Add ice and sparkling water. For added color, add pomegranate seeds.

MAKES 1 SERVING

Appendix A:
Extended Keto-Green Food Lists

Here are two food lists. The first lists the foods you'll choose on the 10-Day Quick Start, and it can double as a shopping list. The second is a comprehensive list I compiled to help you choose the most alkaline and low-carb, ketogenic foods as you go forward. It is organized to help you identify the degree of alkalinity and acidity in common whole foods, as well as their carb content. Please note that just because a food is alkaline, it is not necessarily low in carbs. Remember to eat mostly alkaline low-carb foods in preference to acidic ones.

The 10-Day Quick Start Food and Shopping List

Alkaline Vegetables That Detoxify Estrogen

Broccoli
Brussels sprouts
Cabbage
Cauliflower

Other Alkaline Vegetables

Alfalfa sprouts
Asparagus, green
Avocado (I know, it's a fruit ☺)
Bamboo shoots
Bell peppers
Carrots
Celery
Cucumber
Eggplant
Greens: beet greens, lettuces, kale, spinach, chard, and so forth
Jalapeño
Kimchi
Mushrooms
Onions
Scallions

Seaweed: all types, including nori
Snow peas
Tomatoes
Yellow squash
Zucchini

Protein Choices

Eggs and egg yolks, organic and cage-free
Goat cheese
Organic chicken and turkey
Organic grass-fed beef
Pancetta or bacon (nitrate/nitrite free)
Protein powder, including vegetarian protein powder, such as pea and rice protein (choose one with less than 3 g sugar per serving)
Shellfish: shrimp, scallops, or oysters
Tofu, miso, or tempeh (see vegan swaps on page 77)
White fish, such as sea bass

Liver-Detoxifying Foods and Herbs

Artichoke hearts
Onions, garlic, and scallions
Oregano
Rosemary
Sage
Thyme

Other Quick Start Foods

Bone broth
Vegetable or alkaline broth

Oils and Vinegars
Apple cider vinegar (unfiltered)
Avocado oil

Coconut oil
MCT oil
Olive oil, extra-virgin
Organic ghee or butter (from grass-fed cows)
Rice or coconut vinegar
Sesame oil
Walnut oil

Herbs and Spices

Allspice
Basil, fresh or dried
Bay leaves
Black pepper, ground
Chives, fresh
Cilantro
Cinnamon sticks
Dry mustard
Garlic powder
Ginger root, fresh
Lemons for seasoning
Limes for seasoning
Mint, fresh or dried
Paprika
Parsley, fresh or dried
Red pepper flakes
Sea salt
Tarragon, fresh or dried

Nuts and Seeds

Almond or cashew butter
Almonds
Chia seeds
Flaxseeds
Pistachios
Sesame seeds

Sunflower seeds

Walnuts

Teas

Chai

Chamomile

Cinnamon

Green

Mushroom

Additional

Almond flour

Capers

Coconut aminos

Coffee

Full-fat whipping coconut cream

Kalamata olives

Maca, powdered, or Mighty Maca Plus

Nutritional yeast

Red curry sauce

Roasted red peppers, jarred

Sour cream, light

Tahini

Tamari sauce, preferably low-sodium

Alkaline Food List

Vegetables

Highly Alkaline/Low-Carb Vegetables

Beet greens

Cucumber

Kelp and other sea vegetables

Maca

Parsley

Radishes (black)
Spinach
Sprouts, all types
Vegetable broth

Highly Alkaline/Moderate-Carb Vegetables

Dandelion greens
Jicama
Kale
Turnip greens

Moderately Alkaline/Low-Carb Vegetables

Arugula
Asparagus
Bamboo shoots
Basil
Broccoli
Cauliflower
Celery
Chives
Collard greens
Endive
Green cabbage
Lettuce
Mustard greens
Peppers (hot)
Pumpkin
Radishes (red, white)
Savoy cabbage
Spring greens
Tomato
Turnips
Watercress
White cabbage

Moderately Alkaline/Moderate-Carb Vegetables

Artichoke
Garlic
Green beans
Okra
Soybeans
Squash (winter)

Moderately Alkaline/High-Carb Vegetables

Butter beans
Corn
Ginger
Lentils
Parsnips

Mildly Alkaline/Low-Carb Vegetables

Bell peppers
Bok choy
Brussels sprouts
Eggplant
Herbs and spices
Kohlrabi
Mushrooms
Pickles (not sweetened)
Squash (summer)
Zucchini

Mildly Alkaline/Moderate-Carb Vegetables

Beets
Carrots
Leeks
Onions (red, white)
Peas
Red cabbage
Rhubarb
Rutabaga

Mildly Alkaline/High-Carb Vegetables

Jerusalem artichokes
New baby potatoes
Potatoes with skin
Sweet potatoes
Water chestnuts
Yams

Fruits

Highly Alkaline/Moderate-Carb Fruits

Cantaloupe
Melons, other
Watermelon

Highly Alkaline/High-Carb Fruits

Dried dates and figs
Grapes
Mango
Papaya

Moderately Alkaline/Low-Carb Fruits

Berries
Carob

Moderately Alkaline/Moderate-Carb Fruits

Apricot
Avocado
Lemon
Lime

Moderately Alkaline/High-Carb Fruits

Apple
Banana
Cherries (sour)
Currants

Dates and figs, fresh
Kiwis
Kumquats
Nectarines
Oranges
Passionfruit
Pears
Pineapple, fresh
Raisins
Tamarind
Tangerines

Mildly Alkaline/Low-Carb Fruits
Coconut, fresh
Olives

Mildly Alkaline/Moderate-Carb Fruits
Grapefruit

Mildly Alkaline/High-Carb Fruits
Pomegranate

Nuts and Seeds

Highly Alkaline/Low-Carb Nuts and Seeds
None

Moderately Alkaline/Low-Carb Nuts and Seeds
Chia seeds
Hemp hearts

Mildly Alkaline/Low-Carb Nuts and Seeds
Almond butter
Almond milk
Almonds
Brazil nuts

Pine nuts
Sesame seeds

Fats and Oils

(Note: There are no high- or moderate-carb fats/oils.)

Moderately Alkaline Fats and Oils
Flaxseed oil

Mildly Alkaline Fats and Oils
Avocado oil
Coconut oil
Fish oil
MCT oil
Olive oil, extra-virgin
Sesame oil

Grains

(Note: There are no high- or moderately alkaline grains.)

Mildly Alkaline/High-Carb Grains
Buckwheat
Millet

Flesh Foods and Protein

(Note: There are no high-alkaline flesh foods and protein.)

Moderately Alkaline/Low-Carb Flesh Foods and Protein
Beef juice (a juice extracted from meat through heat)
Bone meal

Condiments

(Note: Carbs in condiments are negligible.)

Moderately Alkaline Condiments
Sea salt
Tamari
Vinegar

Mildly Alkaline Condiments
Mayonnaise, homemade
Nutritional yeast

Acid Food List

Vegetables

Moderately Acid/Low-Carb Vegetables
Tomatoes, canned
Vegetables such as beans or spinach, canned

Moderately Acid/Moderate-Carb Vegetables
Peanuts

Moderately Acid/High-Carb Vegetables
Potatoes with no skin

Mildly Acid/High-Carb Vegetables
Dried beans and peas

Fruits

Moderately Acid/High-Carb Fruits
Fruits, canned in sugar

Mildly Acid/High-Carb Fruits

Cranberries

Nuts and seeds

Plums

Prunes

Mildly Acid/Low-Carb Nuts and Seeds

Cashews

Coconut, dried

Macadamias

Pecans

Pistachios

Pumpkin seeds

Sunflower seeds

Walnuts

Fats and Oils

Moderately Acid Fats and Oils

Grapeseed oil

Sunflower oil

Mildly Acid Fats and Oils

Animal fats

Organic butter

Grains

Highly Acid/High-Carb Grains

Flour, wheat or white

Rice, white

Moderately Acid/High-Carb Grains

Cream of wheat

Kamut

Oats

Rice, brown and basmati
Wheat products

Mildly Acid/High-Carb Grains

Amaranth
Barley
Bran
Bulgur
Cornmeal
Rye
Spelt

Flesh Food and Protein

Highly Acid/Low-Carb Flesh Food and Protein

Beef
Buffalo/bison
Chicken
Eggs, large, organic, and cage-free
Lamb
Pork
Rabbit
Turkey
Venison

Moderately Acid/Low-Carb Flesh Food and Protein

Fish
Shellfish

Condiments

Moderately Acid Condiments

Ketchup
Mayonnaise, commercial
Mustard

Miscellaneous

Moderately Acid/Low-Carb
Coffee
Tea

Moderately Acid/Moderate-Carb
Wine

Moderately Acid/High-Carb
Chocolate

Mildly Acid/Low-Carb
Protein powder (depends on brand)
Yogurt, unsweetened

Appendix B:
Self-Tests

As I explained in Chapter 2, the following self-tests will help you assess your hormonal baseline. Taking the time to administer them will make sure you aren't overlooking anything as you begin this program. Testing yourself again one month after you start, and then again in two months, will show you your progress.

Hormonal Review of Symptoms Checklist

Look at each symptom, listed in the far-left column. Then rate each symptom on a scale from 0 to 3 (0 = no symptoms; 1 = mild; 2 = moderate; 3 = severe). Record your rating in the far-right column under Symptom Score.

Compare your Symptom Score with what is going on with your hormones. For example, let's say you rated your hot flashes as a 3 (severe). Checking the Hormone Relationship column, you see that your estrogen levels may be going up or down (↑ ↓ E); your progesterone levels are declining (↓ P); and your testosterone levels are declining too (↓ T).

Date_____

SYMPTOM	HORMONE RELATIONSHIP	SYMPTOM SCORE
Anxiety	↑E ↓P ↓T ↑C↓TH	
Arthritis	↓T ↓P	
Bladder symptoms	↓E ↓T	
Breakthrough bleeding	↓P	
Breast tenderness	↑E ↓P	
Constipation	↓TH	
Cramps or painful periods	↓P ↑P	
Decreased ability to play sports	↓T ↓TH	
Decreased enjoyment of life	↑E ↓P ↓T	
Decreased sex drive	↑↓E ↓P ↓T↑↓C ↓TH	

SYMPTOM	HORMONE RELATIONSHIP	SYMPTOM SCORE
Decreased strength or endurance	↓T ↓TH	
Decreased work performance	↓E ↓T ↓P ↓TH	
Depression	↑↓P ↑C ↓E ↑↓T ↓TH	
Dry skin/hair	↓E ↓TH	
Fatigue	↑P ↓TH ↓↑T ↑↓C ↑↓E	
Fibrocystic breasts	↑E ↓P	
Fluid retention	↑E ↓P	
Hair loss	↑T ↑↓TH ↑↓E ↑↓P ↑C	
Harder to reach climax	↓T ↓E ↓P	
Headaches	↑↓E ↑↓P ↓T ↑C ↓TH	
Heavy/irregular menses	↑E ↓P	
Hot flashes	↑↓E ↓P ↓T	
Irritability	↑E ↑↓P ↑T ↓C	
Loose stools	↑C ↑TH	
Loss of memory	↑↓E ↑↓P ↓T ↑C ↓TH	
Mood swings	↑E ↓P	
Night sweats	↑↓C ↓E	
Sleep disturbance	↑↓T ↓P ↓E ↑C	
Stomach pain	↑↓C	
Vaginal dryness	↓E ↓T	
Weakness, muscular	↓T ↓P	
Weight gain	↑E ↓P ↓TH	
Weight loss	↑C ↑TH	

Key: E = estrogen / P = progesterone / T = testosterone / C= cortisol / TH = thyroid

Record your total points: _____

Medical Symptom Toxicity Questionnaire

Using the point scale below, rate each of the following symptoms based upon your symptoms over the last thirty days. For each symptom category, total your points.

Finally, add up the totals from each category to come up with your grand total.

POINT SCALE

0 = Never or almost never have the symptom

1 = Occasionally have it; the effect is not severe

2 = Occasionally have it; the effect is severe (it interferes with my life)

3 = Frequently have it; the effect is not severe

4 = Frequently have it; the effect is severe

DIGESTIVE TRACT	HEAD	MOUTH/THROAT
Nausea or vomiting	Headaches	Chronic coughing
Diarrhea	Faintness	Gagging, need to clear throat
Constipation	Dizziness	Sore throat, hoarseness, loss of voice
Bloated feeling	Insomnia	Swollen/discolored tongue, gums, lips
Belching or passing gas	Total: ___	
Heartburn		Canker sores
Intestinal/stomach pain		Total: ___
Total: ___		
EARS	HEART	NOSE
Itchy ears	Irregular or skipped heartbeat	Stuffy nose
Earaches, ear infections	Rapid or pounding heartbeat	Sinus problems
Drainage from ear	Chest pain	Hay fever
Ringing in ears, hearing loss	Total: ___	Sneezing attacks
Total: ___		Excessive mucus formation
		Total: ___
EMOTIONS	JOINTS/MUSCLES	SKIN
Mood swings	Pain or aches in joints	Acne
Anxiety, fear, or nervousness	Arthritis	Hives, rashes, or dry skin
Anger, irritability, or aggressiveness	Stiffness or limitation of movement	Hair loss
Depression	Pain or aches in muscles	Flushing or hot flashes
Total: ___	Feeling of weakness or tiredness	Excessive sweating
	Total: ___	Total: ___

ENERGY/ACTIVITY	LUNGS	WEIGHT
Fatigue, sluggishness	Chest congestion	Binge eating/drinking
Apathy, lethargy	Asthma, bronchitis	Craving certain foods
Hyperactivity	Shortness of breath	Excessive weight
Restlessness	Difficulty breathing	Compulsive eating
Total: ___	Total: ___	Water retention
		Underweight
		Total: ___
EYES	**MIND**	**OTHER**
Watery or itchy eyes	Poor memory	Frequent illness
Swollen, reddened, or sticky eyelids	Confusion, poor comprehension	Frequent or urgent urination
Bags or dark circles under eyes	Poor concentration	Genital itch or discharge
	Poor physical coordination	Total: ___
Blurred or tunnel vision (does not include near- or farsightedness)	Difficulty in making decisions	
	Stuttering or stammering	
Total: ___	Slurred speech	
	Learning disabilities	
	Total: ___	

Scoring

OPTIMAL	MILD TOXICITY	MODERATE TOXICITY	SEVERE TOXICITY
< 10	10–50	50–100	> 100

The Eve Questionnaire

This questionnaire aims to assess your sexual and pelvic health. Once you know your starting number (from 0 to 70; lower is better), it's much easier to track your progress as you change your diet and implement lifestyle changes. Read through each question, and check off your response. (Many of the questions refer to symptoms with sex; if you're not sexually active, answer "never" or give your best guess.)

1. Do you lack energy?
   ☐ Never
   ☐ Some of the time
   ☐ Quite often
   ☐ Always

2. Do you find yourself making up excuses to avoid having sex?
   ☐ Never
   ☐ Some of the time
   ☐ Quite often
   ☐ Always

3. Do you find yourself sexually undesirable?
   ☐ Never
   ☐ Some of the time
   ☐ Quite often
   ☐ Always

4. Is the thought of sex distressing for you?
   ☐ Never
   ☐ Some of the time
   ☐ Quite often
   ☐ Always

5. Do you have discomfort during or after sex?
   ☐ Never
   ☐ Some of the time
   ☐ Quite often
   ☐ Always

6. Is vaginal or vulvar dryness troublesome?
   ☐ Never
   ☐ Some of the time
   ☐ Quite often
   ☐ Always

7. Would you consider yourself frustrated about your sex life?
   ☐ Never
   ☐ Some of the time
   ☐ Quite often
   ☐ Always

8. Do you find it very difficult to become aroused?
   ☐ Never
   ☐ Some of the time
   ☐ Quite often
   ☐ Always

9. Do you lose urine when you cough or sneeze?
   ☐ Never
   ☐ Some of the time
   ☐ Quite often
   ☐ Always

10. Do you use pads or panty liners due to urine leakage?
    ☐ Never
    ☐ Some of the time
    ☐ Quite often
    ☐ Always

SCORING

Review your answers. For every "Never," assign 0 points. For every "Some of the time," assign 3 points. For every "Quite often," assign 5 points. For every "Always," assign 7 points.

Record your total points: _____

Interpretation

If you scored between 0 and 10, you are doing extremely well. Your desire is healthy and intact, with normal vaginal and orgasmic function. But if you scored closer to 15, you may be experiencing some symptoms that could worsen over time, unless you take steps to improve them.

If you scored between 15 and 30, you are having a few arousal, vaginal health, and orgasmic functioning issues that are standing in the way of vibrant sexual health and vitality. Making lifestyle changes now will begin to lower your score.

If you scored between 31 and 50, your lack of interest in and low enjoyment of sex may be due to a number of factors—vaginal pain problems, arousal issues, or urinary problems, among others. But these are all reversible with the right lifestyle changes.

If you scored above 50, your interest in sex, your ability to become aroused, vaginal pain, or other sexual health issues are interfering with the quality of your sex life and pelvic health. These problems, though discouraging, can be improved or completely resolved with proper lifestyle actions, consistently followed.

Positivity Self-Assessment Questionnaire

With this assessment, you can see how your moods respond to the natural approach in a quick and fun way. Record your feelings (as well as information about your menstrual flow and libido) at least weekly, according to the directions. You'll be surprised that in as soon as one month, you'll feel much better emotionally.

Scoring

In the boxes below, rate your moods according to these scores.

0 = Not at all

1 = Minimal

2 = Some

3 = Extremely

Also, on the dates you score your moods, note your menses too. Record one of the following letters under the date:

S = Spotting

L = Light flow

M = Average

H = Heavy

For sexual activity, draw a smiley face ☺ under the date.

DATE ☺	I AM HAPPY AND JOYFUL.	I AM CONTENT.	I AM ENERGETIC.	I AM PRODUCTIVE.	I AM SOCIAL AND FRIENDLY.	I AM ALERT; MY MIND IS FOCUSED.	I FEEL GOOD ABOUT MY BODY.

Daily Tracker

Week Starting _____

Height _____ Weight _____ Waist _____ Hips _____

	MONDAY	TUESDAY	WEDNESDAY	THURSDAY	FRIDAY	SATURDAY	SUNDAY
Intentions:							
Grateful for:							
Cheer word:							
Connected with:							
Oxytocin activity:							
**Joyful							
**Content							
**Energetic							
**Productive							
**Friendly							
**Focused							
**Body love							
Weight:							
Hours of sleep:							
pH:							
Ketones:							
Water intake:							
MM/B/ACV*:							
Bowel movement:							
Physical activity today:							
Why today was great:							

* MM = Mighty Maca Plus, B = baking soda, ACV = apple cider vinegar

Appendix C: Resources

Clinical Laboratories

23andMe: Ancestry and Health

Precision Analytics: Urinary Testing for Hormones, Nutrition and Estrogen Detoxification

Genova Diagnostics: Nutrition testing, Hormones, Estrogen, Detoxification Pathways

Diagnostics Solutions Laboratory: GI-MAP (stool test)

Cyrex Labs: Gluten-Associated Cross-Reactive Foods and Food Sensitivity (Array 4) and Permeability (Array 2)

Ubiome.com: Jane Test (a vaginal health test)

Cell Science Systems: Alcat Food Sensitivity Test

Diagnostechs: Adrenal Stress Index

Quicksilver Scientific: quicksilverscientific.com for Heavy Metals Testing

UltaLabTests.com/drannacabeca (for my recommended blood panels)

Recommended Test Strips and Where to Get Them

Keto PH Test Strips: dranna.com

Hydrion pH Paper: amazon.com

KETO-MOJO Blood Ketone and Glucose Testing Meter Kit or Precision Xtra Blood Ketone Test Strips: amazon.com

Nutritional Supplements

Dr. Anna Cabeca's Mighty Maca Plus

Dr. Anna Cabeca's Keto-Alkaline Detox Support

Dr. Anna Cabeca's Keto-Alkaline Protein Shake (0 g sugar)

Dr. Anna Cabeca's Keto-Green All-in-One Protein Shake Meal Replacement (0 g sugar)

Dr. Anna Cabeca's Optimal Balance (hormone-balancing herbal formula)

Dr. Anna Cabeca's Better Brain and Sleep (magnesium L-threonate)

Hormone support: Vida Optimal Balance; Femquil by Xymogen

Vital-Zymes chewable digestive enzymes by Klaire Labs

Probiotics: Probio ENT, chewable probiotic by Xymogen; Probio Max
Spore-containing probiotics: Thrive probiotic; Megasporebiotic
    by Microbiome Labs
Opti-Lean Fiber from xymogen.com
Argentyn Silver

High-Quality Multivitamins and Nutraceutical Companies

xymogen.com
designsforhealth.com
thorne.com
quicksilverscientific.com for liposomal glutathione
standardprocess.com

Natural Solutions for Women with Vaginal Dryness

Dr. Anna Cabeca's Julva feminine cream
Dr. Anna Cabeca's Pura Balance PPr cream
Good Clean Love natural lubricants
Yes brand natural lubricants
Ayurvedic ghee

Prescription Solutions for Women with Vaginal Dryness

Estrace
Estring
Intrarosa
Vagifem
Prometrium
For compounding pharmacies see PCCARX.com

Kitchenware and Cooking Tools

NutriBullet and Veggie Bullet (love these!)
Vitamix
Hamilton Beach Set 'n Forget Slow Cooker (it is free of lead,
    which many slow cookers contain)
Radiant Life 14-Stage Biocompatible Water Purification System
Ceramic skillets
Cast-iron skillets
Wusthof knives

CorningWare
Glass ovenware, like Pyrex
Bamboo cutting boards
Glass jars and storage bowls

Cosmetics and Beauty Products
Toothpaste by Primal Life Organics
Skincare by Annmarie Gianni
DIY lube and makeup remover
Beautycounter
The Spa Dr.
Mito Q

Chemical-Free Feminine Products
Lotus liners and reusable pads
Organic tampons, liners, and pads

Nontoxic Household Products
EC3 laundry detergent, mold cleaner, and cleaning products
White vinegar
Thieves Oil cleaning products
Seventh Generation

Pest Control
Boric acid tablets

Water Filters
Vollara.com (living water sink system and laundry system)
United Distributors, Inc. (whole-house systems and reverse osmosis)
Berkey Water Filter (when under the sink is not possible)
For lead removal, you want to be looking for NSF/ANSI Standard
    53 for pitcher, faucet, countertop, refrigerator, or in-line filters

Air Filters
Vollara FreshAir surround system
Nikken air purifier
Honeywell HPA300

Meditation Products
Heart Math
Muse headband

Helpful Websites
DrAnnaCabeca.com (see dranna.com/resources)
EWG.org for the Environmental Working Group
IFM.org for the Institute of Functional Medicine and Finding a
   Functional Medicine Doctor
hormonesbalance.com for *Cooking for Hormone Balance* with
   Magdalena Wszelaki
drritamarie.com, site for nutritional endocrinology by Ritamarie
   Loscalzo, DC
drmasley.com, site by Steven Masley, MD
drperlmutter.com, site by David Perlmutter, MD, the empowering neurologist
quicksilverscientific.com

Food Sites
VitalChoice.com and CleanFish.com for wild-caught seafood
westerngrassfedbeef.com for grass-fed beef
ThriveMarket.com
PureIndianFoods.com for ghee
EatPilinuts.com for Pili nuts and butters

Links for Forms and Dr. Anna Resources
dranna.com/resources
dranna.com/evequiz
dranna.com/kegelvideo
dranna.com/oxytocinquiz

Miscellaneous
f.lux (computer app)
gunnar.com, truedark.com: Blue-light-blocking eyeglasses
Zen Tech: Blue-light-blocking filters for iPhones

References

Chapter 1: What's Going On with My Hormones?

Chang, H. K. 2015. "A functional Relay from Progesterone to Vitamin D in the immune system." *DNA and Cell Biology* 34: 379–382.

Davis, S. R., et al. 2008. "Dehydroepiandrosterone Sulfate Levels Are Associated with More Favorable Cognitive Function in Women." *The Journal of Clinical Endocrinology & Metabolism* 93: 801–808.

Dudley, P. S., and Buster, J. E. "Alternative therapy: dehydroepiandrosterone for menopausal hormone replacement." *Treatment of the Postmenopausal Woman* (Third Edition), 2007.

Duncan, K. A., editor. 2015. Estrogen Effects on Traumatic Brain Injury: Mechanisms of Neuroprotection and Repair. Cambridge, Massachusetts: Academic Press.

Maki, P. M., and Dumas, J. 2009. "Mechanisms of action of estrogen in the brain: insights from human neuroimaging and psychopharmacologic studies." *Seminars in Reproductive Medicine* 27: 250–259.

Sabatier, N., et al. 2013. "Oxytocin, feeding, and satiety." *Frontiers in Endocrinology* 4: 35.

Shankar, T., et al. 2015. "Progesterone directly up-regulates vitamin D receptor gene expression for efficient regulation of T cells by calcitriol." *Journal of Immunology* 194: 883–886.

Takayanagi, Y., et al. 2008. "Oxytocin receptor-deficient mice developed late-onset obesity." *Neuroreport* 19: 951–955.

Wirth, M. M. 2011. "Beyond the HPA axis: progesterone-derived neuroactive steroids in human stress and emotion." *Frontiers in Endocrinology* 2: 19.

Zhang, H., et al. 2013. "Treatment of obesity and diabetes using oxytocin or analogs in patients and mouse models." PLOS One 8: May 20.

Chapter 2: Where Are You Now? Test, Don't Guess!

Bongiovanni, B. 2009. "Course: PsychoNeuroEndocrinology 2.0; mastering the functional assessment and correction of HPA-T Axis Imbalanced Patients." Atlanta: Sanesco.

Cekic, M., et al. 2011. "Vitamin D deficiency reduces the benefits of progesterone treatment after brain injury in aged rats." *Neurobiology of Aging* 32: 864–874.

Cordina-Duverger, E., et al. 2013. "Risk of breast cancer by type of menopausal hormone therapy: a case-control study among postmenopausal women in France." PLOS One, November 1.

Guennoun, R., et al. "Progesterone and allopregnanolone in the central nervous system: response to injury and implication for neuro protection." *The Journal of Steroid Biochemistry and Molecular Biology* 146: 48–61.

Chapter 3: What Is the Hormone Fix?

Anton, S. D., et al. 2013. "Effect of a novel dietary supplement on pH levels of healthy volunteers: a pilot study." *Journal of Integrative Medicine* 11: 384–388.

Brinton, R. D. 2008. "Estrogen regulation of glucose metabolism and mitochondrial function: therapeutic implications for prevention of Alzheimer's disease." *Advanced Drug Delivery Reviews* 60: 1504–1511.

Caciano, S., et al. 2015. "Effects of dietary acid load on exercise metabolism and anaerobic exercise performance." *Journal of Sports Science & Medicine* 14: 364–371.

Davis, E. 2018. Ketogenic diet plan. Ketogenic diet resource. Online: ketogenic-diet-resource.com/ketogenic-diet-plan.html.

Dawson-Hughes, B., et al. 2008. "Alkaline diets favor lean tissue mass in older adults." *The American Journal of Clinical Nutrition* 87: 662–665.

Dawson-Hughes, B., et al. 2009. "Treatment with potassium bicarbonate lowers calcium excretion and bone resorption in older men and women." *The Journal of Clinical Endocrinology & Metabolism* 94: 96–102.

Devine, A., et al. 1995. "A longitudinal study of the effect of sodium and calcium intakes on regional bone density in postmenopausal women." *The American Journal of Clinical Nutrition* 62: 740–745.

Frassetto, L., et al. 2001. "Diet, evolution and aging—the pathophysiologic effects of the post-agricultural inversion of the potassium-to-sodium and base-to-chloride ratios in the human diet." *European Journal of Nutrition* 40: 200–213.

Frassetto, L., et al. 2005. "Long-term persistence of the urine calcium-lowering effect of potassium bicarbonate in postmenopausal women." *The Journal of Clinical Endocrinology & Metabolism* 90: 831–834.

Groos, E., et al. 1986. "Intravesical chemotherapy. Studies on the relationship between pH and cytotoxicity." *Cancer* 58: 1199–1203.

Hahn, T. J., et al. 1979. "Disordered mineral metabolism produced by ketogenic diet therapy." *Calcified Tissue International* 24: 17–22.

Heaney, R. P., et al. 2003. "Calcium absorption varies within the reference range for serum 25-hydroxyvitamin D." *Journal of the American College of Nutrition* 22: 142–146.

Konner, M., et al. 2010. "Paleolithic nutrition: twenty-five years later." *Nutrition in Clinical Practice* 25: 594–602.

Lindeman, R. D., and Goldman, R. 1986. "Anatomic and physiologic age changes in the kidney." *Experimental Gerontology* 21: 379–406.

Masino, S. A., and Rho, J. M. 2012. "Mechanisms of ketogenic diet action." In Jasper's Basic Mechanisms of the Epilepsies [Internet]. 4th edition.

Murakami, K., et al. 2008. "Association between dietary acid-base load and cardiometabolic risk factors in young Japanese women." *British Journal of Nutrition* 100: 642–651.

Paoli, A., et al. 2014. "Ketogenic diet in Neuromuscular and Neurode-generative diseases." *BioMed Research International*, July 3.

Park, H. M., Heo, J., and Park, Y. 2011. "Calcium from plant sources is beneficial to lowering the risk of osteoporosis in postmenopausal Korean women." *Nutrition Research* 31: 27–32.

Raghunand, N., et al. 1999. "Enhancement of chemotherapy by manipulation of tumour pH." *British Journal of Cancer* 80: 1005–1011.

Robey, I. F., and Nesbit, L. A. 2013. "Investigating mechanisms of alkalinization for reducing primary breast tumor invasion." *BioMed Research International*, July 10.

Schwalfenberg, G. K. 2009. "Improvement of chronic back pain or failed back surgery with vitamin D repletion: a case series." *Journal of the American Board of Family Medicine* 22: 69–74.

Schwalfenberg, G. K. 2012. "The alkaline diet: is there evidence that an alkaline pH diet benefits health?" *Journal of Environmental and Public Health*. Epub, October 12.

Sebastian, A., et al. 2003. "Estimation of the net acid load of the diet of ancestral preagricultural Homo sapiens and their hominid ancestors." *The American Journal of Clinical Nutrition* 76: 1308–1316.

Sebastian, A., and Morris, R. C. 1994. "Improved mineral balance and skeletal metabolism in postmenopausal women treated with potassium bicarbonate." *New England Journal of Medicine* 330: 1776–1781.

Tabatabai, L. S., et al. 2005. "Arterialized venous bicarbonate is associated with lower bone mineral density and an increased rate of bone loss in older men and women." *The Journal of Clinical Endocrinology & Metabolism* 100: 1343–1349.

University of Pennsylvania School of Medicine. 2017. "Timing meals later at night can cause weight gain and impair fat metabolism: Findings provide first experimental evidence of prolonged delayed eating versus daytime eating, showing that delayed eating can also raise insulin, fasting glucose, cholesterol, and triglyceride levels." *ScienceDaily*, June 2.

Vormann, J., et al. 2001. "Supplementation with alkaline minerals reduces symptoms in patients with chronic low back pain." *Journal of Trace Elements in Medicine and Biology* 15: 179–183.

Welch, A. A., et al. 2013. "A higher alkaline dietary load is associated with greater indexes of skeletal muscle mass in women." *Osteoporosis International* 24: 1899–1908.

Wigglesworth, V. B. 1924. "Studies on ketosis: I. the relation between alkalosis and ketosis." *Biochemical Journal* 18: 1203–1216.

Zofková, I., and Kancheva, R. L. 1995. "The relationship between magnesium and calciotropic hormones." *Magnesium Research* 8: 77–84.

Chapter 4: Getting Started

Balunas, M. J., et al. 2008. "Natural products as aromatase inhibitors." *Anticancer Agents in Medicine and Chemotherapy* 8: 646–682.

Catenacci, V. A., et al. 2016. "A randomized pilot study comparing zero-calorie alternate-day fasting to daily caloric restriction in adults with obesity." *Obesity* 24: 1874–1883.

Dennehy, C., and Tsourounis, C. 2010. "A review of select vitamins and minerals used by postmenopausal women." *Maturitas* 66: 370–380.

Editor. 2017. "Groundbreaking study on healing leaky gut with the strains used in Just Thrive Probiotic." Just Thrive, online: thriveprobiotic.com.

Gunn, C. A., et al. 2015. "Increased intake of selected vegetables, herbs and fruit may reduce bone turnover in post-menopausal women." *Nutrients* 7: 2499–2517.

Hahn, T. J., et al. 1979. "Disordered mineral metabolism produced by ketogenic diet therapy." *Calcified Tissue International* 24: 17–22.

Hodges, R. E., and Minich, D. M. 2015. "Modulation of metabolic detoxification pathways using foods and food-derived components: A scientific review with clinical application." *Journal of Nutrition and Metabolism,* June 16.

Kamal, P. 2018. "Maca; Summary of maca." Examine.com, June 14.

Lucas, M., et al. 2009. "Effects of ethyl-eicosapentaenoic acid omega-3 fatty acid supplementation on hot flashes and quality of life among middle-aged women: a double-blind, placebo-controlled, randomized clinical trial." *Menopause* 16: 357–366.

Marinac, C. R., et al. 2016. "Prolonged nightly fasting and breast cancer prognosis." *JAMA Oncology* 2: 1049–1055.

Mattson, M. P., Longo, V. D., and Harvie, M. 2017. "Impact of intermittent fasting on health and disease processes." *Ageing Research Reviews* 39: 46–58.

Nair, P. M., and Khawale, P. G. 2016. "Role of therapeutic fasting in women's health: An overview." *Journal of Midlife Health* 7: 61–64.

Tucker, K. L., et al. 2006. "Colas, but not other carbonated beverages, are associated with low bone mineral density in older women: The Framingham Osteoporosis Study." *The American Journal of Clinical Nutrition* 84: 936–942.

Wang, Y., et al. 2016. "Curcumin in treating breast cancer: a review." *Journal of the Association for Laboratory Automation* 21: 723–731.

Zajac, A., et al. 2014. "The effects of a ketogenic diet on exercise metabolism and physical performance in off-road cyclists." *Nutrients* 6: 2493–2508.

Zinedine, A., et al. 2006. "Review on the toxicity, occurrence, metabolism, detoxification, regulations and intake of zearalenone: an oestrogenic mycotoxin." *Food and Chemical Toxicology* 45: 1–18.

Chapter 7: Protect Yourself from Toxic Overload and Hormone Disruptors

Berk, M., et al. 2013. "So depression is an inflammatory disease, but where does the inflammation come from?" *BMC Medicine* 11: 200.

Chandrasekaran, V. R., Hsu, D. Z., and Liu, M. Y. 2014. "Beneficial effect of sesame oil on heavy metal toxicity." *Journal of Parenteral and Enteral Nutrition* 38: 179–185.

Darbre, P. D., and Harvey, P. W. 2014. "Parabens can enable hallmarks and characteristics of cancer in human breast epithelial cells: a review of the literature with reference to new exposure data and regulatory status." *Journal of Applied Toxicology* 34: 925–938.

Dodson, R., et al. 2012. "Endocrine disruptors and asthma-associated chemicals in consumer products." *Environmental Health Perspectives* 120: 935–943.

Falk, R. T., et al. 2013. "Relationship of serum estrogens and estrogen metabolites to postmenopausal breast cancer risk: a nested case-control study." *Breast Cancer Research* 15: R34.

Gao, X., et al. 2017. "Gestational zearalenone exposure causes reproductive and developmental toxicity in pregnant rats and female offspring." *Toxins* 9: 21.

Garcia-Nino, W. R., and Pedraza-Chaverrie, J. 2014. "Protective effect of curcumin against heavy metals–induced liver damage." *Food and Chemical Toxicity* 69: 182–201.

Kalagatur, N. K., et al. 2015. "Antagonistic activity of Ocimum sanctum L. essential oil on growth and zearalenone production by Fusarium gramminearum in maize grains." Frontiers E-Book.

Lovelace, C.E.A., and Nyathi, C. B. 1977. "Estimation of the fungal toxins, Zearalenone and aflatoxin, contaminating opaque maize beer in Zambia." *Journal of the Science of Food and Agriculture* 28: 288–292.

Maragos, C. M. 2010. "Zearalenone occurrence and human exposure." *World Mycotoxin Journal* 3: 369–383.

Partanen, H. A., et al. 2010. "Aflatoxin B1 transfer and metabolism in human placenta." *Toxicological Sciences* 113: 216–225.

Saito, R., et al. 2017. "Aryl hydrocarbon receptor induced intratumoral aromatase in breast cancer." *Breast Cancer Research and Treatment* 161(3): 399–407.

Sang, Y., Li, W., and Zhang, G. 2016. "The protective effect of resveratrol against cytotoxicity induced by mycotoxin, zearalenone. *Food & Function* 7: 3703–3715.

Santen, R. J., Yue, W., and Wang, J. P. 2015. "Estrogen metabolites and breast cancer." *Steroids* 99 (Pt A): 61–66.

Taylor, K. W., et al. 2018. "Associations between personal care product use patterns and breast cancer risk among white and black women in the Sister Study." *Environmental Health Perspective,* February 21.

Zinedine, A., et al. 2007. "Review on the toxicity, occurrence, metabolism, detoxification, regulations and intake of zearalenone: an oestrogenic mycotoxin." *Food and Chemical Toxicology* 45: 1–18.

Chapter 8: Stop Stress from Stressing You Out

Beck, T. 2012. "Estrogen and female anxiety." *The Harvard Gazette,* August 9.

Bergland, C. 2013. "The neuroscience of post-traumatic stress disorder; neuroscientists have discovered specific brain areas linked to PTSD." *Psychology Today,* November 5.

Boundless Biology. Course: "The Light-Dependent Reactions of Photosynthesis." Online: courses.lumenlearning.com/boundless-biology /chapter/the-light-dependent-reactions-of-photosynthesis/.

Chevalier, G., et al. 2012. "Earthing: health implications of reconnecting the human body to the Earth's surface electrons." *Journal of Environmental and Public Health.* Epub, January 12.

do Amaral, J. A., et al. 2015. "The effects of musical auditory stimulation of different intensities on geometric indices of heart rate variability." *Alternative Therapies in Health and Medicine* 21: 16–23.

Graziano, P. 2010. "In a mouse model relevant for PTSD, selective brain steroidogenic stimulants (SBSSs) improve behavioral deficits by normalizing allopregnanolone biosynthesis." *Behavioural Pharmacology* 21: 438–445.

He, S., et al. 2014. "Job burnout, mood state, and cardiovascular variable changes of doctors and nurses in a children's hospital in China." *ISRN Nursing,* March 9.

HuaLin, C., et al. 2018. "Pregnenolone-progesterone-allopregnanolone pathway as a potential therapeutic target in first-episode antipsychotic-naïve patients with schizophrenia." *Psychoneuroendocrinology* 90: 43–51.

Keating, C., et al. 2013. "Effects of selective serotonin reuptake inhibitor treatment on plasma oxytocin and cortisol in major depressive disorder." *BMC Psychiatry* 13: 124.

Marx, C. Presentation. "Neurosteroids in PTSD and Co-occurring Conditions Biomarkers to Therapeutics." NCpsychiatry Online: ncpsychiatry .org/assets/2017AnnualMeeting/Handouts/OnePage/2._neurosterioids _in_ptsd_and_co-occuring_conditions-christine_marx.pdf.

McFarlane, A. C. 2010. "The long term costs of traumatic stress: intertwined physical and psychological consequences." *World Psychiatry* 9: 3–10.

McNamee, D. A., et al. 2009. "A literature review: the cardiovascular effects of exposure to extremely low frequency electromagnetic fields." *International Archives of Occupational and Environmental Health* 83: 919–933.

Melcangi, R. C., and Panzica, G. C. 2014. "Allopregnanolone: state of art." *Progress in Neurobiology* 113: 1–5.

Miller, G. E., et al. 2002. "Chronic psychological stress and the regulation of pro-inflammatory cytokines: A glucocorticoid-resistance model." *Health Psychology* 21: 531–541.

Resnick, E. M., Mallampalli, M., and Carter, C. L. 2012. "Current challenges in female veterans' health." *Journal of Women's Health* 21: 895–900.

Robinson, M. 2016. "Exploring transition factors among female veterans of Operation Enduring Freedom/Operation Iraqi Freedom." Dissertation: Walden University.

Rouen, P. A. 2009. "Study of Women Veterans in Menopause." Dissertation: University of Michigan.

Sabatier, N., et al. 2012. "Oxytocin, feeding, and satiety." *Frontiers in Endocrinology* 4: 35.

Sanders, R. 2014. "New evidence that chronic stress predisposes brain to mental illness." *Berkeley News,* February 11.

Shanafelt, T. D., Sloan, J. A., and Habermann, T. M. 2003. "The well-being of physicians." *The American Journal of Medicine* 114: 513–519.

Sunkaria, R., Kumar, V., and Saxena, S. C. 2010. "A comparative study on spectral parameters of HRV in yogic and non-yogic practitioners." *International Journal of Medical Engineering and Informatics* 2: 1–14.

Vaudry, H., and Tsutsui, K. 2013. "Neurosteroids: Relationship between BDNF and Allopregnanolone in corticlimbic neuron." Frontiers ebook.

Zhang, H. F., et al. 2015. "Electro-acupuncture improves the social interaction behavior of rats." *Physiology & Behavior* 151: 485–493.

Chapter 9: Vaginal Health: Get Your Sexy Back

Archer, D. F., et al. 2017. "Comparison of intravaginal 6.5mg (0.50%) prasterone, 0.3mg conjugated estrogens and 10μg estradiol on symptoms of vulvovaginal atrophy." *The Journal of Steroid Biochemistry and Molecular Biology* 174: 1–8.

Bazi, T., et al. 2016. "Prevention of pelvic floor disorders: international urogynecological association research and development committee opinion." *International Urogynecological Journal* 27: 1785–1795.

Chiechi, L. M., et al. 2003. "The effect of a soy rich diet on the vaginal epithelium in postmenopause: a randomized double blind trial." *Maturitas* 45: 241–246.

Copas, P., et al. 2001. "Estrogen, progesterone, and androgen receptor expression in levator ani muscle and fascia." *Journal of Women's Health & Gender-Based Medicine* 10: 785–795.

Davis, R., and Parish, S. 2015. "Testosterone in women: can the challenges be met?" *The Lancet* 3: 588–590.

Editor. 2017. "Endoceutics Fact Sheet: Dyspareunia: Genitourinary Syndrome of Menopause (GSM) and Vulvovaginal Atrophy (VVA)." Retrieved from endoceutics.com/hormones-health/dyspareunia-gsmvva.

Fede, C., et al. 2016. "Hormone receptor expression in human fascial tissue." *European Journal of Histochemistry* 60: 2710.

Glaser, R., and Dimitrakakis, C. 2013. "Reduced breast cancer incidence in women treated with subcutaneous testosterone, or testosterone with anastrozole: a prospective, observational study." *Maturitas* 76: 342–349.

Glaser, R., and Dimitrakakis, C. 2014. "Rapid response of breast cancer to neoadjuvant intramammary testosterone-anastrozole therapy: neoadjuvant hormone therapy in breast cancer." *Menopause* 21: 673–678.

Glaser, R., and Dimitrakakis, C. 2015. "Testosterone and breast cancer prevention." *Maturitas* 82: 291–295.

Helwick, C. 2014. "Testosterone/anastrozole implants relieve menopausal symptoms in breast cancer survivors." *The ASCO Post,* October 15.

Ke, Y., Gonthier, R., and Labrie, F. 2017. "Impact of sample extraction on the accurate measurement of progesterone in human serum by liquid chromatography tandem mass spectrometry." *Journal of Chromotography* 1052: 110–120.

Khandelwal, S. 2017. "Early age at menopause: How should we empower them with health." *Maturitas* 100: 190.

Manson, J. E., et al. 2017. "Menopausal hormone therapy and long-term all-cause and cause-specific mortality." *JAMA* 318: 927–938.

Margery, L. S., et al. 2013. "Management of symptomatic vulvovaginal atrophy." 2013 position statement of the North American Menopause Society. *Menopause* 20: 888–902.

Morgentaler, A., et al. 2015. "Testosterone therapy and cardiovascular risk: advances and controversies." *Mayo Clinic Proceedings* 90: 224–251.

Younes, J., et al. 2017. "Women and their microbes: the unexpected friendship." *Trends in Microbiology* 26: 16–32.

Zethraeus, N., et al. 2017. "A first-choice combined oral contraceptive influences general well-being in healthy women: a double-blind, randomized, placebo-controlled trial." *Fertility and Sterility* 107: 1238–1245.

Chapter 10: Rejuvenate Your Routine: Movement and Sleep

Cheema, B. S., et al. 2015. "The feasibility and effectiveness of high-intensity boxing training versus moderate-intensity brisk walking in adults with abdominal obesity: a pilot study." *BMC Sports Science, Medicine and Rehabilitation* 7: 3.

Jorge, M. P., et al. 2016. "Hatha yoga practice decreases menopause symptoms and improves quality of life: a randomized controlled trial." *Complementary Therapies in Medicine* 26: 128–135.

Lancel, M., et al. 2003. "Intracerebral oxytocin modulates sleep-wake behaviour in male rats." *Regulatory Peptides* 114: 145–152.

Lu, Y. H., et al. 2016. "Twelve-minute daily yoga regimen reverses osteoporotic bone loss." *Topics in Geriatric Rehabilitation* 32: 81–87.

Robinson, K. M. 2013. "10 surprising health benefits of sex." WebMD .com.

Santoro, N., et al. 2011. "The SWAN song: study of women's health across the nation's recurring themes." *Obstetrics and Gynecology Clinics of North America* 38: 417–423.

Xie, L., et al. "Sleep drives metabolite clearance from the adult brain." *Science* 342: 373–377.

Chapter 11: Master Your Most Important Hormone, Oxytocin

Brody, S. 2002. "High-dose ascorbic acid increases intercourse frequency and improves mood: a randomized controlled clinical trial." *Biological Psychiatry* 15: 371–374.

Liu, H., et al. 2016. "Is sex good for your health? A national study on partnered sexuality and cardiovascular risk among older men and women." *Journal of Health and Social Behavior* 57: 276–296.

Matchock, R. L. 2015. "Pet ownership and physical health." *Current Opinion in Psychiatry* 28: 386–392.

Michael, Y. L., et al. 1999. "Health behaviors, social networks, and healthy aging: cross-sectional evidence from the Nurses' Health Study." *Quality of Life Research* 8: 711–722.

Ormsby, S. M., and Smith, C. A. 2016. "Evaluation of an antenatal acupuncture intervention as an adjunct therapy for antenatal depression (AcuAnteDep): study protocol for a pragmatic randomised controlled trial." *Trials* 17: 93.

Taylor, S. E., et al. "Relation of oxytocin to psychological stress responses and hypothalamic-pituitary-adrenocortical axis activity in older women." *Psychosomatic Medicine* 68: 238–245.

Acknowledgments

Writing a book is a dream come true from when I was a teenager (though then, to be honest, I wanted to write a romantic, sexy novel!). I am so grateful to be accomplishing this dream now, and I have many people to thank and acknowledge. Being brief is hard, but I'll give it my best try.

First, I want to acknowledge my children, Brittany, Amanda, Amira, Garrett (in heaven), and Avamarie, all of whom have been at my side all along the way. I am so grateful to have your love and light in my life. You have also given me strength to keep looking for more medical answers and to never give up. This extra effort has been worth it for us all and so many others.

I want to thank my mother, Claire Suidan Cabeca, who both in life and in death was an inspiration and mentor. She always told me that education is something no one could ever take away from me, and she pressed me to always seek answers and keep learning. She also always said travel is one of the best forms of education, and she was sure right about that—my travels have opened my eyes and heart in ways no book has or could have done.

My father, Bill, passed away at ninety-one but for my whole life was such a strong influence. I try to live by his wisdom: "Try to understand each other, get along, and never go to bed angry."

I am truly grateful for my extended family, near and far, especially for my brother John, who has always emphasized and lived out another family motto, "If there is something to be done, just do it!"; for my brother Robert, who perseveres gracefully; and for my dearest, crazy cousin Grace, who has been such a big blessing and support to me throughout our lives. Grace, you are my sister. To Sarah, Jamy, and my goddaughter, Izzy, I so love you girls.

I am grateful for the strong matriarchs in my lineage: especially my mother; my tauntes Helen and Elsa; and my taunte Simone, who, widowed young, raised her family of four as a single mom with grace, strength, and kindness and showed me that family (and laughter) takes precedence.

I am grateful to my dear friends who have unconditionally supported me in my goals and on my journey: Dr. Angeli Akey, Dr. Ellie Campbell, Mary Butin, Dr. Bobbi Davanzo, and my childhood friends Yael Vilenski and Helene Burke, who always encouraged my dreams. And to Shiroko Sokitch, MD; Mikell Parsons, DC; Rebecca Davis, and Robin Nielsen for your endless support and love.

It's my pleasure to acknowledge—very gratefully—all my work family, the team of people who have been at my side, often working endlessly on one of my new missions or latest ideas, and who always have kept my vision to spread healing, love, and connection at the front of their own efforts. Thank you so much to Jamellette Difoot for your constant love and prayers, you are a second momma to us all, to Lori Thomas for your dedication and care, to Jamy Casiano and David Gomes for always being there to help others, to Jessica Baxter for your kind care of our clients and expert chef and recipe help, to Rossana Alvarado for your exuberance and generosity always, and to Amanda Brayman for your essential assistance. Thank you, Shibani Subramanya and Josh Koerpel, for your genius, dedication, and guidance, and Chris Loch for your eloquent creativity. Diane Blum, thank you for all the years of helping me get my thoughts and ideas on paper. You have all contributed to the betterment of lives of women and families in such beautiful ways. Thank you for your support and care of me too while I focused on this manuscript, and your dedication to our clients and customers.

There are so many educators and influencers that have been in my life who have really inspired me, including those from my ob-gyn residency and training at Emory University, as well as my dear colleagues and friends Steven Masley, MD; J. J. Virgin; Magdalena Wszelaki; Dr. Jessica Drummond; Lara Briden, ND; Alan Christianson, ND; David Scheiderer, MD; and profound educators Jeffrey Bland, PhD; David Perlmutter,

MD; and Dr. Christiane Northrup, whose book *Women's Bodies, Women's Wisdom* was given to me by a patient in 2000. I hope my book, like hers, will open the eyes of more patients and physicians as they work together to heal holistically to their best abilities.

I will be forever grateful to my agent, Heather Jackson, and collaborator, Maggie Greenwood, who have made my dream become a reality, and to my editor, Marnie Cochran, for all her work and patience with me. Indeed, to the whole Ballantine Books and Penguin Random House teams—I thank you.

Finally, I would like to express my utmost heartfelt and sincerest gratitude to all my patients and clients, who throughout the decades have inspired me to be a better doctor and healer. Thank you for sharing your lives, stories, and trust with me. Please keep believing in your innate ability to heal, and pass these lessons on.

Index

About the Author

ANNA CABECA, DO, OBGYN, FACOG, is an internationally acclaimed menopause and sexual health expert, global speaker, and pioneering promoter of women's health. She is Emory University–trained and triple-board certified in gynecology and obstetrics, integrative medicine, and antiaging and regenerative medicine, and is the creator of the Hormone Fix, a diet and holistic lifestyle program for menopausal women.

Her areas of specialty include bioidentical hormone treatments and natural hormone-balancing strategies, and she has received extensive acclaim for her virtual transformational programs including Women's Restorative Health, Sexual CPR, and Magic Menopause. She created the successful and popular alkaline superfoods drink Mighty Maca PLUS, and a top-selling, rejuvenating feminine vulvar cream for women, Julva.

She was named 2018 Innovator of the Year by Mindshare, the number one conference for health and wellness influencers, and was also honored with the prestigious 2017 Alan P. Mintz Award, presented annually by the Age Management Medicine Group to the most outstanding physician who displays clinical excellence and entrepreneurship.

Dr. Cabeca has reached hundreds of thousands of women around the globe, inspiring them to reclaim their optimal health and realize they can journey through menopause and find more purpose and pleasure than they ever dreamed possible. She has been interviewed by all major television networks and has been featured in *InStyle, The HuffPost, First,* and *MindBodyGreen.* She balances her passion for women's health with faith, grace, and skill, while raising her four daughters on St. Simons Island, Georgia, and leading the nonprofit foundation she created in honor of her son, Garrett V. Bivens, who tragically died as a toddler.

Follow her journey on her blog at dranna.com

About the Type

This book was set in Minion, a 1990 Adobe Originals typeface by Robert Slimbach (b. 1956). Minion is inspired by classical, old-style typefaces of the late Renaissance, a period of elegant, beautiful, and highly readable type designs. Created primarily for text setting, Minion combines the aesthetic and functional qualities that make text type highly readable with the versatility of digital technology.